BLACK GIRLS BREATHING

BLACK GIRLS BREATHING

HEAL FROM TRAUMA, COMBAT CHRONIC STRESS, AND FIND YOUR FREEDOM

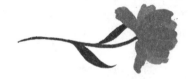

JASMINE MARIE

balance

New York Boston

Balance
Hachette Book Group
1290 Avenue of the Americas
New York, NY 10104
GCP-Balance.com
@GCPBalance

First Edition: December 2024

Balance is an imprint of Grand Central Publishing. The Balance name and logo are registered trademarks of Hachette Book Group, Inc.

The publisher is not responsible for websites (or their content) that are not owned by the publisher.

The Hachette Speakers Bureau provides a wide range of authors for speaking events. To find out more, go to hachettespeakersbureau.com or email HachetteSpeakers@hbgusa.com.

Balance books may be purchased in bulk for business, educational, or promotional use. For information, please contact your local bookseller or the Hachette Book Group Special Markets Department at special.markets@hbgusa.com.

Print book interior design by Marie Mundaca

Library of Congress Cataloging-in-Publication Data
Names: Marie, Jasmine, author.
Title: Black girls breathing : heal from trauma, combat chronic stress, and
     find your freedom / Jasmine Marie.
Description: First edition. | New York : Balance, [2024] | Includes index.
Identifiers: LCCN 2024025123 | ISBN 9781538756621 (hardcover) |
     ISBN 9781538756645 (ebook)
Subjects: LCSH: African American women—Health and hygiene. | African
     American women—Mental health. | Psychic trauma. | Mind and body therapies. |
     Self-realization.
Classification: LCC RA564.86 .M27 2024 | DDC 616.85/210082—dc23/eng/20240711
LC record available at https://lccn.loc.gov/2024025123

ISBNs: 978-1-5387-5662-1 (hardcover); 978-1-5387-5664-5 (ebook)

Printed in Canada

MRQ

Printing 1, 2024

To Mom:
Thank you for your sacrifices.
I love you dearly.

CONTENTS

WRITE THE VISION. MAKE IT PLAIN.

GROWING UP, SUNDAYS were for church. For my family, the day felt like a beacon of light, a source of restoration, and a reward for making it through the heaviness of the week. The heaviness came from us kids being "an only" at school and the microaggressions my parents experienced at work. They felt the taxation of trying to ensure their Black children would have as many opportunities as possible when they were older by signing them up for after-school activities in their youth: orchestra, dance, choir, and private piano lessons. The weight of the old adage "twice as good, half as much" motivated my parents to keep striving for the sake of their children in spite of their fatigue.

My mom shouldered most of the domestic responsibilities, even while working full-time. She made sure all the kids were fed, had finished their homework, and were excelling at their extracurricular activities. She rarely complained, but the heaviness of day-to-day life, managing all her responsibilities, and creating more opportunities for her kids than she'd had growing up was written on her face and carried in her body. She just needed to make it to Sunday. Then her cup would be refilled and her hope renewed for the week ahead, before the ins and outs of her daily life would empty her cup again.

Those early experiences showed me the power of spaces that act as a refuge for Black bodies. What we would feel, experience, and witness in church for those two-plus hours on Sunday mornings would affirm and encourage us in ways the world never could. Here, we were safe and seen. Here, we envisioned futures of brighter tomorrows, worshipped with joy, and had our hope restored.

The power of beginning each week with a ritual in a restorative space was planted deep into my psyche and Spirit long before I birthed black girls breathing.® I was practicing affirmations in church before I even knew to call them that; in church, these affirmations came in the form of call-and-response singing and reading scriptures. One verse that would fuel me with courage and faith to call forth things that didn't yet exist was Habakkuk 2:2: "Write the vision; make it plain."

If you grew up in the Black church, you've heard this affirmation before. It shows up often in hymns and popular worship songs. The lyrics would state the verse over *mm-hmms* and *that's rights*. "Write the vision; make it plain." And the choir or congregation would affirm the possibility with an *it is so* or *amen*. The pastor or choir would repeat this phrase over and over, and the church would emphatically affirm it until it was felt across the congregation—resonating deep in our bones. The feeling of assuredness that everything would be all right, no matter the tribulations of the week, would settle in my Spirit.

The internal pull to write a vision and make it plain led me to bring the breathwork that had been essential to my own healing journey back to my community after completing my breathwork training. Breathwork soothed my nervous system in response to emotional triggers, healed my body from the effects of past trauma, and eased the physical symptoms I was experiencing as a result of chronic stress and anxiety. I didn't see tools like these commonly used in my community despite the clear need for them, given the well-documented physical and emotional ailments experienced by the Black community as a result of all the obstacles we faced in the world. So, I wrote the vision: a world where Black women could live full, thriving lives. And I made it plain: using breathwork as a tool to address their trauma and heal their bodies.

Black girls breathing® was born of that vision. Since 2019, we have gathered in person and virtually. Both the name and the intention were inspired by how restored I felt at church on Sunday mornings growing up; our sunday balm® community was launched to continue this work in deeper ways in 2023. We use the breath to surface the buried emotions and energy housed in the body while witnessing each other's journeys and sharing our struggles and experiences in a world where we seldom feel safe. Through my work with black girls breathing,® I've provided free access to the tool of breathwork for tens of thousands (with a goal of reaching one million). With the breath, I've guided Black women to trust their bodies and all that they discover therein. I've witnessed the surfacing of harrowing traumas and the beauty of many women's journeys as they come out of the darkness of their wounds to emerge on the other side. I've seen firsthand how stress shows up specifically in Black bodies and how our particular stressors respond to the breath. I've gained a wealth of knowledge from the many participants my work has touched, and I have made history bringing this work to global platforms and audiences, proudly representing Black women whenever I have the opportunity.

Those Sunday mornings at church continued to bear fruit in my young-adult years. The launch of black girls breathing® was my response to the deep need for Black bodies to find refuge from the world. If freedom wasn't fully available to us, it was my intention that for those ninety minutes, or however long we were together, we would have a safe space to refill our cups and feel seen and heard, just as I'd experienced at church. This book is an offering that further extends that invitation.

As you read the words that have made it from my heart and mind to the page, I encourage you to engage with the topics and the journey of introspection and healing with an open heart and self-compassion. I hope that you emerge wiser and more self-assured and hopeful than you were before as you experiment with the many tools and exercises included within this offering—sinking deeper into your body and tapping in to the radical wisdom contained within.

I crafted each chapter to bring awareness to common themes I've observed in facilitating this work for many Black women. (But as Black women are not a monolith and we encompass many experiences and identities, it would be impossible to detail them all within one book. My intention is that these themes are a good starting point and catalyst for your healing so you can apply these concepts however they resonate for you.) You can start your own journey with this book on the first page or skip around to the themes and chapters that speak to your healing needs the most. There may be many moments when the content feels heavy, when it resonates but makes you feel triggered. I invite you to take a step back, offer yourself some nurturing, tender care (tuning in to a rest practice or soothing exercise in the book) as you navigate through the topic and reflect on your own truths, and then pick up the book again whenever you're ready. Allow yourself to feel deeply and explore, while also caring for your body's needs. Keep in mind that in spite of any resistance you might experience, *your body is strong enough to feel, process, and witness any pain that's ready to be released.*

In case no one has already told you this today, I love you. And I am so, so glad you're here. Thank you for entrusting me with being a part of your beautiful healing journey. It is an honor that I do not take for granted. And I hope that through your own healing, you will write the vision of the possibilities for your life and make it plain.

With the deepest breath,
Jasmine Marie

Chapter 1

CHRONIC STRESS IS OUR CRISIS

IN EARLY 2014, my stress levels reached heights I had never experienced before. I was constantly at the doctor's office with a new physical symptom that, after further examination, the doctor would affirm was due to stress. I was one year postgraduation from NYU Stern and working in global brand marketing as part of a fast-track leadership development program at the second-largest global consumer goods company in the world. The program was meant to take undergraduate graduates and, in three years, put them on the same career trajectory as an MBA graduate with five to six years of work experience. Along with the demands of the global projects I was leading and collaborating on as a twenty-three-year-old recent grad, I was also in a relationship with a narcissistic partner. My body was operating in fight-or-flight mode all the time, which was normalized in the culture of "success over everything" at a top business school and corporation based in NYC. Consistent sleep was hard to come by when my stress levels soared, and I always brought work home with me since my primary concern during the week was to stay on top of all my projects. I had no concept of boundaries when it came to my work or my romantic relationships, and my self-esteem and health suffered because of it. Chronic stress led to more bouts of depression and anxiety, creating a never-ending cycle. My personal story and experience with chronic stress is reflected in many other Black women's experiences. I know I'm not alone in that. My personal and professional experiences to date have allowed me to bear intimate witness to the damage that stress has on our ability to have a thriving, full, and healthy life.

Throughout this book, you will be invited to deepen your inhales. This isn't just a relaxation exercise or some kind of woo-woo experience. It's a direct weapon against the high cortisol levels wreaking havoc in our bodies due to chronic stress. A symbolic call-and-response, if you will, urging us to address the stress that might otherwise build up and contribute to our early deaths.[1] The stress doesn't stop at spiking our cortisol levels, but causes other physical and mental ailments. In the United States, Black women are more likely to die from breast cancer, heart disease, stroke, and ovarian cancer than any other demographic.[2] Underpaid, underresourced, and the sickest demographic in our nation,

---

1   Jolaade Kalinowski, Heather Wurtz, Madeline Baird, and Sarah S. Willen, "Shouldering the Load Yet Again: Black Women's Experiences of Stress During COVID-19," *Mental Health* 2 (December 2022), www.sciencedirect.com/science/article/pii/S2666560322000809.

2   Jillian McKoy, "Racism, Sexism, and the Crisis of Black Women's Health," *The Brink*, October 31, 2023, www.bu.edu/articles/2023/racism-sexism-and-the-crisis-of-black-womens-health.

Black women are robbed of the quality of life that our ancestors dreamed we would have.

This likely isn't the first time you've seen stats indicating that we're more stressed out than any other demographic. But something tells me that in this particular season of your life, you picked up this book ready for change and seeking practical tools, a new outlook, and a healthier way of coping with traumas to create a new way forward. The first step to any long-term change is awareness of the problem. And though the realities presented in this chapter are hard to swallow, looking these truths directly in the face will give us the clarity to understand what we are up against and find the tools to combat them.

A LEADING CAUSE OF STRESS: THE STRONG BLACK WOMAN ARCHETYPE

What I witnessed while building the black girls breathing® community reaffirmed to me that at the root of much of our stress was the deeply ingrained belief, reinforced generation after generation, that we had to be strong. The Strong Black Woman, or SBW, is what I'll sometimes call her. You may identify with her characteristics. The Strong Black Woman has to be perfect. She shows up for everyone in her life, including colleagues, family, and friends, and she does so cheerfully, without a complaint (at least not expressed directly to them). Notably, the Strong Black Woman doesn't consider herself to be part of the equation when she makes many of the decisions in her daily life. To do something for herself would be considered selfish, not only by her, but also by her boss, her friends, and her extended family, all of whom have learned to judge her against an impossible standard. With those external environments shaping her life experience, she has internalized these pressures and expectations.

Deep, deep down, she believes things like *It is selfish to consider myself. Saying no is selfish. Who do I think I am to prioritize myself?* She knows that if she doesn't meet everyone's expectations, she will become the subject of familial gossip at the next holiday dinner, or she will be excluded from consideration for the next promotion. This deep-seated fear keeps her constantly showing up for others, no matter how badly she is neglecting herself. Even as we observe these thought patterns in our own lives, we need to extend grace to ourselves. After all, we didn't learn to operate this way on our own. The SBW archetype was handed down to us Black women through societal and familial conditioning.

We can find the archetype's roots in slavery, when Black women were expected to play the role of "the mammy"—the mother figure tending to her master's children. She nursed and raised them, while her own children would never get the privilege of knowing her in that way. Her body was not her own. Survival depended on her ability to ensure that everything flowed with ease in the house during the day, while she was subject to the master's lustful urges at night. Long after emancipation, oppression still grips the lives of Black women today.

The Strong Black Woman's nervous system is taxed; chronic stress is her norm. The joy of bringing life into this world is coupled with the sobering reality that she is five times more likely to die while giving birth than her white counterparts.[3] Her depression and anxiety make her irritable, fatigued, and angry. Growing up, she was not given any tools to address her mental health other than praying about it or recognizing that her concerns were "not that bad" compared to others who had it worse, implying that she should be grateful and push through any problems. Perversely, overextending herself brings her comfort. It reinforces the belief that if she can help others, then her problems aren't that bad. She loses herself in the roles of employee, mother, daughter, sister, granddaughter, niece, family bank account, and breadwinner. However, the minute she begins to experience freedom of any kind, especially financially, she is burdened with the responsibility of reaching back and helping those around her. While her white counterparts may get to use their abundance to plant seeds for their futures, she is obliged to help others in her proximity—often to her detriment—because her community lacks the generational wealth (and infrastructure) for her loved ones to get by without her assistance. She is tired.

By the time Black women are introduced to my work, they are often at their wits' end. They feel foggy and uncertain, and they know something has to change, but they don't have the slightest clue where to start. They are executives, midlevel career women, and hourly workers experiencing similar workplace traumas regardless of their position and title. They are unemployed and weighed down by the belief that they are failing, coupled

---

3   Akilah Johnson, "For Some Black Women, the Fear of Death Shadows the Joy of Birth," *Washington Post*, December 14, 2023, www.washingtonpost.com/health/interactive/2023/black-women-pregnancy-mortality-fear.

with the fear that if they fail, and fall, there is no safety net to catch them. Because the Black women I meet are often operating under the subconscious belief that their value is based on their performance, leading them to strive for perfection, they have become disconnected from their bodies and their somatic wisdom. They have become numb to their bodies' cues for hunger, thirst, and sleep. They have locked away all of their innate wisdom in a box, and they are afraid of opening that box and discovering what they might find there.

I teach Black women how to better connect with their bodies and with their breath and to give themselves permission to rest and do nothing. It is a practice that saves lives. Women who've been coming to our black girls breathing® sessions share how long it took them to release the trauma and stress housed in their bodies and nervous systems, to become more attuned to their bodies and their needs and then take the brave next step of honoring those needs. They share how much practice it took to allow themselves to not be so strong. To unravel. To rest and feel comfortable doing nothing after intensive, active breathwork in our sessions. They admit how saddened they become looking at their former selves and how hard it was for them to rest, as rest feels foreign to bodies that have been conditioned to overwork, to bodies that have not belonged to us for centuries and that we still do not feel complete autonomy over.

Hopefully after you've been able to read, sit with, and incorporate the techniques offered in this book, you'll be able to envision a life that doesn't always require you to be strong and have it together, a life in which the idea of continuously operating under the weight of chronic stress feels foreign to you. I hope you give yourself permission to fall apart when life calls for it, knowing you have the tools to put yourself together again when it's time, and to choose many occasions and seasons in life to center yourself and your needs.

SOCIETAL CAUSES OF STRESS

I would be remiss if I didn't address the reality that chronic stress from our external environments permeates our lives as Black women; we would be gaslighting ourselves if we blamed our stress solely on our personal choices. Even when we take steps to reduce our stress, we continue to confront systemic injustices and daily microaggressions that drain our mental, emotional, and physical energy and make us feel as though there is no way out. For example, if you were raised in a neighborhood where a quality education, accessible childcare, and after-school support for youth were unavailable, you might have been exposed to recurring violence and traumatic events that undermined your sense of safety as a child. According to Maslow's hierarchy of needs, safety is essential for healthy human development.[4] Alleviating all those stressors would have required you to leave that neighborhood and seek a quality education elsewhere in order to have a good career. Given that Black women earn only sixty-seven cents for every dollar that white men make, it's extremely difficult for those born

---

4   Saul Mcleod, "Maslow's Hierarchy of Needs," Simply Psychology, January 24, 2024, www.simplypsychology.org/maslow.html.

into poverty or living on the edge of it to extract themselves from those circumstances.[5] In our productivity-driven culture, where we're told to pull ourselves up by our bootstraps, working to shift our situations while already chronically stressed is not a sustainable solution. Although many of us find ourselves in this predicament and muster the miraculous strength to pull ourselves out of these circumstances, this cycle of overwork is contributing to our early deaths.

We are often dismissed by the very systems that our non-Black peers have been encouraged to lean upon for support when they need it, and we are often told that we are overreacting when we speak up. Take our healthcare system, for example. Though so many of us have been conditioned to push through physical and mental pains, by the time we do muster the courage and energy to seek help from a physician, we are often met with disparaging comments that affirm our hesitancy to seek help in the first place. These are comments like "You're probably overreacting." "These symptoms are normal." "I'm not going to refer you for testing. We can just monitor the issue and see what happens." (Can you see how this experience would reinforce the "I'll do it all by myself" Strong Black Woman trope?) Medical discrimination transcends class differences and zip codes. From Serena Williams to the average Black woman, so many of us have stories of not having our health concerns taken seriously or investigated when we bring them up.

---

5   "It's Time to Pay Black Women What They're Owed," National Women's Law Center, July 20, 2023, https://nwlc.org/resource/black-womens-equal-pay-day -factsheet.

This makes me wonder how much more chronic stress we experience because our symptoms are typically dismissed as normal until they can no longer be ignored. If my doctor had taken my stress-induced rashes more seriously, would I have been able to prevent the problem from escalating to a more serious health condition that got triggered by stress later in life? Would earlier testing have helped me take preventative measures against health issues to which I was predisposed? Unfortunately, our chronic stress often goes undiagnosed and undetected by our health system until it's too late.

Predominantly Black neighborhoods are statistically more likely to experience industrial pollution, exposing us to unclean water sources (including lead contamination) and predisposing us to chronic respiratory conditions like asthma.[6] We are also more likely to live in food deserts, where we lack readily available access to fresh food sources. Although we can learn techniques to manage our stress (like the breathwork exercises in this book), how helpful can those techniques be if the air we're breathing is toxic and if we can't find fresh, nonprocessed food within a five-mile radius to nourish our bodies and minds? These social determinants of health perpetuate chronic stress and illness in our society, with sparse public resources to address them. There are far too many factors contributing to the chronic stress epidemic to address them all in this book, but I'll touch on many common experiences for Black women to raise awareness and

---

6 "What to Know About Lead Exposure and Poisoning in Black Communities," Medical News Today, November 10, 2023, www.medicalnewstoday.com/articles /history-of-lead-poisoning-in-black-communities.

provide you with the tools to understand and address the complexities of these issues.

ADDRESSING OUR CHRONIC STRESS WITH THE BREATH

When I experienced unexplainable health episodes, followed by multiple doctor's visits, I distinctly recall an appointment during which a doctor said, "It seems like you're stressed. How can you reduce your stress? Well, never mind—everyone's stressed." It was as if she were about to help me come up with some solutions until she remembered that making it in the city meant enduring, not curing, stress. It was simply a normal part of a New Yorker's life. At that point, I knew I needed more than just my usual therapy sessions to help me deal with the stress that was wreaking havoc on my life. I knew exactly where my stress was coming from and could analyze its impact, but my mind was tired, and my body desperately needed relief.

The church I attended in Harlem helped ground me on the weekends, before the Sunday scaries took over, so I decided to get even more involved. Volunteering at the church's new community center led me to my first breathwork class. It was taught by my pastor's personal breathworker, who was an older Black woman. I vividly remember my experience after that session. It was the first time in a long time that I had space to think. My worries about work and my personal life no longer felt as pressing and urgent. There was space in my body to breathe. My chest didn't feel so tight. My face relaxed. I was able to be more present in the moment rather than function on autopilot. After my first experience with the breath, I began to consider questions like these: What can I let go of because it is causing so much stress in my life? What duties and "other people's stuff" have I been carrying as though they are mine to address? I began to incorporate consistent breathwork classes into my life and reflect more deeply.

Make no mistake—no major changes were happening in my external world amid these revelations. In fact, pressures at work grew even worse. I continued to experience the ups and downs of being in a relationship with a narcissistic partner. But I was experiencing noticeable changes within me. Those internal shifts would later expand into my outside world and influence how I related to others and set boundaries to bring forth my best self.

I describe breathwork as an active form of meditation, meaning that this tool requires your participation and is more rigorous than a relaxing, mindful meditation that focuses solely on calming your mind and observing your body's resting state and thoughts. With intentional breaths, following various sequences and rhythms depending on the specific breathwork pattern, this tool activates your parasympathetic nervous system, which governs the "rest and digest" function and helps your body respond to high cortisol levels and stress. If your nervous system is constantly operating in fight-or-flight mode, it is overtaxed and does not have the capacity to calm the mind and body in response to daily stressors (much less traumatic experiences). With consistent breathwork practice, you can train your nervous system like a muscle to respond to triggers, and you can become your own best advocate in navigating stressful situations.

> The vagus nerve is the largest component of the
> parasympathetic nervous system, the part of the nervous
> system that governs our "rest and digest" function.[7]

The history of breathwork can be traced back to American indigenous cultures and is also foundational to yoga and Indian cultures. Given the generational knowledge I've witnessed in my practice and the somatic tools used by my ancestors, I suspect that this wisdom is also part of African cultures. As many African cultures relied on oral tradition, there is not a lot of physical documentation of these practices. But our ability to use our bodies to heal ourselves is familiar to many in the African diaspora. As you explore and experiment with the various breathwork and somatic tools described in this book, know that this work is not entirely foreign to your DNA. You have the innate wisdom to heal your body.

THE TRUTH ABOUT UNRAVELING OURSELVES FROM CHRONIC STRESS

The mainstream message that's been sold to us suggests that healing ourselves means that everything in our lives will be perfect. When this expectation of perfection is met by a harsher reality, we may feel that something is wrong with us or that we're doing healing all wrong. But I want to be real with you: disentangling ourselves,

7   Jessica Migala, "7 Ways to Stimulate Your Vagus Nerve and Why It Matters," Everyday Health, December 27, 2023, www.everydayhealth.com/neurology/ways-to-stimulate-your-vagus-nerve-and-why-it-matters.

our lives, and our beliefs from all that we knew when chronic stress was our norm will feel like experiencing a slow death many times on the journey of unlearning and healing. Your perception of reality will shift drastically and then begin to leak into your external actions. Your sense of self, your values, and your relationships—all of those foundational components of your identity—will be massively altered, and sis, it will feel unsettling. I want to affirm that it is normal to experience anger, regret, shame, and extreme sadness in the process. There is nothing wrong with you. When you allow yourself to unravel from the Strong Black Woman archetype and other limiting identities, you begin to reposition yourself in the world in ways that don't require you to function in an exhausted state. It is an act of courage to challenge beliefs and deeply embedded patterns that are actually detrimental. I am so proud of you for embarking on this difficult but rewarding journey that few are willing to take, and I'm grateful to have the opportunity to accompany you down this path.

IDENTIFYING THE MAJOR STRESSORS IN YOUR LIFE

As you prepare to take a deeper dive into the healing practices in this book, I invite you to first reflect on the areas in your life where stress is taking a toll on you.

Work and Professional Stress

Whether you're in the process of getting your undergraduate or graduate degree or navigating the complexities of climbing the corporate ladder, as a Black woman, you will experience microaggressions in the workplace and at school. The label "micro" is misleading, given that being on the receiving end of a microaggression is anything but small. As we continue to break glass ceilings when it comes to representation in various industries and obtain certain positions, we occupy spaces that aren't prepared for our brilliance and often haven't addressed the discrimination lurking within office politics and procedures. Something as seemingly minor as what is considered an appropriate hairstyle in the workplace can be discriminatory. Yes, we are breaking barriers, but oftentimes being among the first or one of the only comes at the expense of our overall health. If you can recount a time when you were subjected to a micro- or macro-aggression by a non-Black person in the workplace, I'd wager that the impact on your mind and body outlasted the moment it happened. Maybe you didn't even realize it was an offense until afterward, when you were able to sit with your discomfort around what transpired. The uneasiness you felt in your body lingered, and you likely replayed the episode over and over again in your mind, trying to make sense of it all. And you likely engaged in this mentally exhausting activity while continuing to interact with the same people who caused the offense, doing your best work, and perhaps outperforming everyone else on your team. Can you see how that stress that our society describes as micro has compounding effects? We generally encounter more than one microaggression in the workplace per day, but each one has a multiplying effect like an ongoing trauma that needs to be addressed (more on trauma in the next chapter).

Downplaying the effects of this kind of stress can lead you to pile on more to your schedule than is actually healthy for you and to convince yourself that "it's not that bad" and that you don't need to look for employment elsewhere (perhaps in a hybrid office environment or hourly gig-economy position that limits micro-aggressions). Dismissing these incidents entirely can lead to burn-out that impacts your ability to work. When I've seen this happen to other Black women, I always encourage them to take what-ever time off is possible to just rest and/or leave that environment behind, even temporarily, to give them the space to come up with a plan, as not retreating from these offenses will have a serious impact on their health.

Home and Environmental Stress

Whether you're in a relationship, married, or single, whether you live by yourself or with roommates in the city or suburbs or on a farm, decreasing the stressors in your home life is important because your home is your "safe space." We retreat to our homes to pour into ourselves, find our footing, and recenter before we go back out into the world. While the outside world can be full of surprises, the ideal home environment contains as few stressors as possible.

Observing how you feel in your home and your neighbor-hood and investing in making them a safe refuge is important. Do you like where you live? Do you feel safe? If not, what can you do to improve your environment if moving is not possible right now? Can you spend more time getting to know your neighbors

BLACK GIRLS BREATHING

and finding a trusted few who can check in on you or look out for your space? If you live in a predominantly non-Black neighborhood and feel othered, can you minimize the potential for unpleasant encounters by getting recommendations for grocery stores, restaurants, and social spaces from people you trust or opting to order online? If you live with others and experience stress because of an unequal distribution of labor in the home, have the necessary conversations to divide the work more equally, creating a schedule and assigning tasks. If household chores are a source of stress and you can afford to outsource the work from time to time, perhaps you can order groceries online, hire a cleaner, or pay for a laundry service. I'm not advocating that you become a hermit, but I want you to know that just because many of the older women in our lives have accomplished these tasks day in and day out, and just because we're used to doing them, doesn't mean that they don't add to our stress levels. We also don't live in the same society as our elders. As we seek to reduce stress in our day-to-day lives, it's imperative we make the necessary adjustments in our places of refuge.

Financial Stress

Money and the stress around it are not just individual problems but also generational ones for our community. As Black women's earnings increase, rarely are we able to enjoy the fruits of our own labor. Due to the financial disparities and a lack of generational wealth in the Black community, when we advance, we tend to have to reach back to pull up our families and those around us, unlike

16

many of our peers whose parents' and grandparents' privilege have enabled them to create generational wealth. Few in the Black community know the peace of having someone in our family to catch us if we make a financial misstep. As a result, the perceived and actual lack of money in our community creates a wealth of stress. Shouldering not just our own financial burdens but also those of the people closest to us may lead us to stay in unhealthy work environments and overwork because we are concerned about how our financial standing or lack thereof will impact those around us. Although we may be accustomed to offering financial support to our families, it is essential that we set clear boundaries around how we spend money on ourselves (spending more on higher priorities) and how we share our resources with others (having clear guidelines on how much we're willing to loan, who we choose to loan to, etc.) in order to decrease financial stress. This reflection may lead you to a new lifestyle that reduces stress. Maybe you no longer enjoy living in the city because it is causing you unnecessary headaches. Maybe a longer commute is worth the savings on living expenses. Maybe your shopping habit is causing more stress than happiness so you begin to develop more of a minimalist lifestyle. These are just some examples of where your reflection may lead you as you choose to center your peace over a lifestyle that may be more externally influenced than tied to your personal happiness and values.

As we do this individual work, I want to reiterate that while we can take responsibility for our own actions, we continue to experience inequalities that are beyond our control. Black women continue to be paid less despite being the most educated demographic in the US.[8] These societal factors compound our stress and adversely affect our ability to live healthy lives, so we do what is within our control on an individual level and work collectively to move the needle forward on systemic changes.

Personal and Familial Stress

The people closest to you have a direct impact on your well-being. Decreasing relational stress requires you to remove yourself from codependent relationships that may have felt like the norm and prioritize relationships with family, friends, and partners that are characterized primarily by peace, harmony, and mutual support. (We'll talk more about fostering community care in chapter 5.) Do your closest relationships fill your cup and make you feel seen and heard? Or do you spend a lot of time with people simply because of a sense of obligation—for example, with a childhood friend or cousin you grew up with? You may experience a sense of dread when you spend time (or even think about spending time) with these people. If this is the case for you, how have you normalized pushing through dread and dis-ease? How has investing in unhealthy relationships cultivated a familiarity with, and perhaps an unconscious attraction to, more relationships like these? Examine your closest bonds to locate any major sources of stress.

---

8   Rachaell Davis, "New Study Shows Black Women Are Among the Most Educated Group in the United States," *Essence*, October 27, 2020, www.essence.com /news/new-study-black-women-most-educated.

Identifying those stressors doesn't automatically mean that you have to end those relationships. But if a relationship is unbalanced—perhaps in ways that the other party might not even realize because you've shared this dynamic for so long—practice leaning out in ways that create more ease. This may mean that you're no longer the first person they turn to when they're struggling. Creating a more balanced relationship could also mean doing more things together that bring you joy rather than simply offering them a shoulder to cry on.

Take time to examine your closest relationships and identify where you can implement immediate, practical changes that lessen stressful dynamics.

GO-DEEPER EXERCISE: PRACTICAL WAYS TO DECREASE EXTERNAL STRESSORS

After considering potential sources of stress in this chapter, take a deeper dive into practical ways to begin alleviating these burdens. As we discussed, not all external stressors can be immediately remedied, but it helps to be aware of where your stress is coming from so you are better prepared and consider any changes you might be able to make in the future. Feel free to use the following chart to jot down some of the revelations that surfaced while reading this chapter. I also encourage you to return to this exercise to create a practice of continuously evaluating any major stressors wreaking havoc in your life. Once you're aware of any energy leaks, you can enact a plan to combat them.

Reflective Prompts	Work & Professional	Home & Environmental	Financial	Personal & Familial	Other Sources of Stress:
I notice my body tense when:					
Other mental and emotional indicators that are not helping my overall well-being are:					
In the next week, I can begin moving these things off my plate:					
I may have normalized ____, but I'm willing to unlearn and create a new normal that reduces my daily stress levels.					
I cannot immediately change but will work toward improvement in this area.					

Reflective Prompts	Work & Professional	Home & Environmental	Financial	Personal & Familial	Other Sources of Stress:
I will aim to improve the above in _____ days / weeks / months / years. [circle time metric]					

SITTING STILL: A REST PRACTICE FOR DOING NOTHING

As we explore several somatic practices in this book, with breathwork being the main tool, there will be many opportunities to try active modalities to address the chronic stress housed in your body. However, an equally powerful practice, especially for those of us who are overworked and underappreciated, is the practice of doing nothing. We'll explore several ways for you to indulge in rest in the next chapter, but to prepare, I'd like you to attempt setting aside fifteen minutes of "nothingness." Whether it's when you first wake up in the morning, before you begin an evening routine at night, or right before you take your lunch break or a midday nap, set a timer for fifteen minutes and find a quiet space where you can do absolutely nothing. What I want you to also explore with this exercise is what "doing nothing" means to you. What does doing nothing look and feel like to you? I won't give more instructions than that, as this is an opportunity for you to collect data on where the state of your nervous system might be. This information will help you identify any areas for improvement as we explore and detail some of the difficulties we Black women have with rest in the upcoming chapters. Once you allocate time for this exercise, get curious and answer the following questions. (There are no right or wrong answers. You are responding to these questions in order to use them as data points later on. So, tuck your answers in your back pocket to keep in mind as you continue reading.)

- How did you define "doing nothing" for this activity?
- What were the thoughts that surfaced for you during these fifteen minutes?
- On a scale of one to ten (*one* being extremely uncomfortable and *ten* being extremely comfortable), how comfortable did your body feel during this exercise?

Chapter 2

HEAL THE BODY

THE SAD, OVERWHELMING reality for Black women is that the effects of trauma leak into every aspect of our lives. Beyond the daily stressors we experience in our personal and professional lives, we live in a heightened state of fight or flight that creates continuously high cortisol levels in our bodies. In this traumatized state that is compounded by the generational trauma we may have inherited, we embody what I call the Broken-Down Black Woman. Her nervous system is wrecked, unbeknownst to her, but its effects permeate her entire life. High-level functioning is normal for her but is ultimately killing her. Yet this way of being has been taught and subconsciously passed down to her for generations and generations. In essence, it's all she knows. And sometimes the familiarity of this state makes healing feel too foreign a concept and arduous a task for her.

Trauma is a Greek word that means "wound." Think of a time when you had a physical wound. Maybe as a child you fell off your bike or scraped your knee on the playground. Well after the fall, you were left with a physical injury that was likely painful, tender, and raw, reminding you of that scrape or fall. Maybe you or your caregivers had to take extra care to gently clean, sterilize, and bandage the wound so it would heal properly, and you developed a scab over the once-exposed tissue. The scab, of course, didn't look like your skin before the injury, but it did allow you to at least stop bandaging the wound, and maybe then you felt comfortable returning to your regular childhood activities. After some time, the scab turned into scar tissue, and you were healed physically. However, the incident may have left a mental imprint that made you hesitant (at least initially) to return to the activity that had caused the injury. Perhaps you were afraid of risking another injury, even if you took precautions against it, like wearing kneepads and a helmet to protect you.

This example of a physical wound or trauma is similar to how we experience emotional and psychological traumas. Maybe we've witnessed or directly experienced a traumatic incident that left a lasting imprint on our psyche, impacting the way we think and navigate the world long after the event has passed. It can have such a significant impact on our mental and emotional health that carrying the weight of this burden for long stretches of time morphs into physical disease. Trauma ultimately impacts our brain development. This is the reality of long-standing, unaddressed trauma in our bodies. But how have I seen that trauma show up specifically in us?

By the time the Broken-Down Black Woman finds my work or joins a black girls breathing® breathwork session or our sunday balm® community, she is often dissociated from her body. She's learned to stifle her pain, exhaustion, angst, and unease—leaning in to numbness—so much so that finally having emotional and physical space to unwind creates an avalanche of emotions. Getting her past this moment of overwhelm so she can begin to heal is a journey in and of itself. The trauma has been suppressed for so long that confronting trauma from a previous chapter of her life feels like death.

Emotions and physical sensations related to deeply embedded trauma feel not only foreign but extremely dangerous to her. When I encourage her to engage in practices that surface these emotions and the painful reality of the traumatic situations she's been through, I often get reactions like these:

> *I started to do the journaling and the meditation, but then all these traumas kept coming up one after the other, and I don't think I can handle it. I just keep crying. It's too much.*

> *Thank you for these resources and I appreciate your notes, but I just don't think I'm ready for all of this.*

> *I started the breathwork, but I didn't feel ready to face all of these truths. I realize I've been avoiding so much. Avoiding has kept me feeling safe, though.*

My job then is to gently encourage the exploration of those traumas. I tell her that her body can handle this process, though it might be extremely difficult after hundreds of years of programming to not have ownership of her body and to treat her body like a machine meant only for productivity in service to others. The concept of serving herself with her body is foreign to her and generally unsafe to explore, to say the least. This stage of the healing process is what I call the breakdown before the glow-up, so to speak. It's important not to minimize how difficult and unsettling this part of the process can be.

One would think that introducing breathwork as a new tool, which can be uncomfortable to try, would be the difficult part of the process. But I often see Black women struggling the most with rest, the "doing nothing" portion of a breathwork session (recall your responses to the "doing nothing" exercise in chapter 1). It's not the intensive breaths, the duration of each inhale and exhale, or the time reserved for that active breathing that's difficult; it's being tasked with taking a break from that intensity and permitting themselves to just be in the space that they created. When I reflected deeply on that reality, it made sense. Black women have been programmed to keep pushing beyond their emotional, physical, and mental limits rather than caring for themselves and their bodies. We have this magical ability to exist in extremes without any issues. Detaching our identities from the work we can do and the pain we endure creates something of an identity crisis. Permitting rest is such a foreign concept to Black women that although breathwork can be an uncomfortable new practice, the part they resist is the rest. They'd rather endure the discomfort of intentional slow- or fast-paced breathing than experience the body slowing down and witnessing what arises. The unfamiliarity and discomfort of being still shows up subconsciously when women chime in with comments like these:

What's this song that's playing?

Will we get the playlist and recording?

When's the next session?

The disruption this causes when introducing breathwork got to such a point that I started to preempt any commentary and offer guidelines to ensure that the rest portion of the session would be taken more seriously. I affirmed how uneasy resting could feel. "Doing nothing" went against every fiber of their being and their bodies' conditioning, but it was that important for them to practice experiencing rest. It was important not just to talk about unlearning old patterns but to lean in to what that feels like physically. It's one thing to understand what you need and mentally process the trauma you've endured. It's another thing to embody it.

Healing does not require expensive retreats and self-care products that might be relaxing but don't provide the deep trauma care needed. True healing involves a complete systemic overhaul of how our society has benefitted from the very nature of Broken-Down Black Women. Our society doesn't actually benefit from our healing, from a Black woman recognizing her innate worth and living from that truth. "Oh…she's no longer working herself to the bone for this company that's passed her up for promotions three times?" "What do you mean she now has boundaries and standards for how she wants to be treated by her romantic partner?" "What do you mean, 'no'? You don't have kids. You should be sacrificing yourself for my needs!" Now, of course those sentiments may not be shared aloud, but they are implied and felt. The heavy burden of potentially disappointing others outweighs the deep taxation on this Black woman's body.

It is common for stress in different areas of our lives to be compounded, so the effects and harm leak into our everyday lives. The Broken-Down Black Woman is more prone to experience the unsettling of her nervous system due to a mentally and emotionally abusive relationship because of her people-pleasing conditioning. During the most stressful time in my professional life prior to starting black girls breathing® (because I have since experienced even greater stress), I was also experiencing the ups and downs of a toxic relationship. That relationship left me feeling disconnected from my value, worth, and identity; the relationship's end catalyzed the healing journey that would help birth this work and show me the power of healing the trauma housed in my nervous system. I used the breath to repair my life and strengthen my relationship to myself—learning to trust my own judgments and see clearly my innate value. It is not uncommon for Black women to catalyze their healing in the aftermath of a romantic relationship. A common theme for heterosexual Black women participating in our healing circles and communal dialogue is that when they begin to unpack long-unaddressed trauma, they often find the root of that trauma in a man—either her father / father figure growing up or a man with whom she had a romantic relationship. That realization is both enlightening and deeply painful, as many of us have wanted nothing more in our quest for love and security than to be seen, heard, and protected by our Black men.

INTIMATE TRAUMA

A patriarchal society hurts men as well as women. In our community, the thread of pain and trauma and the emotional avoidance that runs rampant today date back to slavery. Imagine how traumatic events like suddenly being stripped away from their families and being valued solely for their strength and whatever work they could provide affected the way that Black men viewed themselves, the world around them, and partnership—especially with Black women.

It's difficult to have nuanced conversations on social media exploring the depths of trauma in our community and its effects on our relationships. These conversations require an openness to listen, understand, explore, and see multiple perspectives. Although a communal dialogue format can help to dissect, examine, and have robust conversations on this topic, I'm going to try my best to address some of the dynamics that Black men encounter in their relationship with Black women here. The reality is that many Black men in the household are conditioned to see that their sole responsibility as a parent is to provide financially, so they are unable to connect emotionally and vulnerably in romantic relationships. It can be difficult to dive deeper and heal when we have conversations about this in public forums. We want to move beyond clickbait topics like "all Black women hate Black men" and into a space where we can observe how unaddressed and long-held generational traumas and societal norms are creating the relational dynamics that are way too common today. So, as we begin to address this topic in this book, know that healing involves being triggered and facing hard, uncomfortable truths. To heal a thing, we must push ourselves to see that thing clearly, no matter how uncomfortable.

We cannot seek reparations from Western civilizations for the horrors of slavery while also denying the effects of that trauma and the dysfunction it has created in our communities. Unhealthy behaviors don't just appear out of nowhere. There's always a root cause. And as uncomfortable as it feels to address these realities, it is important to do so if we want to heal. And if you're reading this book, you're likely ready for that process and that healing.

Many Black women I've encountered in our healing work have deep childhood father wounds that resulted in low self-esteem and self-worth and made them more prone to unhealthy, unbalanced relationships in their adulthood. Our relationships with our parents and first caregivers shape our identities and what we believe about love when we are children. That serves as the foundation for how we feel about ourselves and what we believe is possible for our lives, including our sense of self-trust, self-love, and self-worth. The subconscious or conscious beliefs about our value that get ingrained in us at an early age shape our relationships and who we'll choose to love as we grow older.

How many women do you know who end up in relationships that feel familiar to them, but from the outside looking in, you cannot understand why they accept gaslighting, noncommitment, and emotional unavailability from their partners when they show up in the world vibrant and a blessing to those around them? As a friend, family member, or confidant, you'll point out how their brilliance stands in stark contrast to their mate. You then see them constantly dimming their light in order to appease and one day "earn" the affection of their significant other. Although these women want to rewrite the story's ending with their romantic partner, they subconsciously and inevitably re-create the dynamics they witnessed in childhood. Maybe her father was emotionally distant and she wants to win over an emotionally unavailable man so the little girl in her is finally seen and chosen. Or maybe her father was in and out of the house, so getting the hot-and-cold, flighty guy to finally commit is what she feels she needs to finally not feel abandoned. The list goes on and on. She doesn't realize that she's trying to right the wrongs she did not create. She's unaware of the strength of these forces and patterns in her life, so she misinterprets that pull she feels in the relationship as home when it's really just more of the same up-and-down dynamics that she's used to. She'll do her best with the chaos in the relationship until she's finally had enough.

By the time this woman comes to black girls breathing,® she's reached her breaking point. She's had enough of intimate relationships filled with trauma—and she is ready to heal. She's fully aware of the impact that trauma has had on her life, and she may have tried therapeutic tools like journaling, reflection, or even talk therapy, but her external world still looks and feels the same. She keeps allowing the same dynamics in her romantic relationships despite the different faces. She finally realizes the healing has to go deeper. She has to address the trauma long held in her cells; thinking through the problem isn't enough, because the damage and beliefs are buried deep in her subconscious.

Though she feels ready for change, she must confront the

reality of how uncomfortable it feels for her body to surface repressed emotions. She'll question if she's ready for such deep pain. And even though I'll affirm to her that she is ready, she'll have to unearth a deeper level of bravery to engage in the process of stripping, unlearning, and breaking down in order to build anew.

It is safe to feel pain in your body.

Your body is strong enough to feel pain.

It is safe to feel these emotions surface in your body.

Because of the Angry Black Woman archetype and being told "Speak when spoken to" and "I'll give you something to cry about" when we were children, we tend to have extremely repressed emotions that over time wreak havoc on the body, leading to both mental and physical diseases. Healing our dysfunction and truly moving toward a thriving and purposeful life filled with inner peace starts with developing greater awareness of our physical body.

MORE ABOUT TRAUMA

The Center for Addiction and Mental Health defines trauma as "a lasting emotional response that often results from living through a distressing event. Experiencing a traumatic event can harm a person's sense of safety, sense of self, and ability to regulate emotions and navigate relationships." There are three main types of trauma: acute, chronic, and complex.

Acute trauma results from a single incident. Chronic trauma results from repeated events or prolonged harm, such as domestic violence or abuse. Complex trauma is exposure to multiple traumatic events.[1]

TAKING OWNERSHIP OF OUR BODIES

The first step to addressing trauma, stress, and anxiety in the body, and creating a better relationship to your body in general, is awareness. As Maya Angelou once said, "When you know better, do better." The deep trauma held by people in the African diaspora is rooted in our history of others having ownership of our bodies. For those of us with enslaved ancestors, our bloodlines have only recently and slowly begun to experience full autonomy.

Let's take some time to think about that. If someone has not been taught or given the tools to tune in to their body, how do they grow into an individual who listens to it, trusts it, and uses its wisdom to make daily decisions to keep it safe and comfortable? How do we get to that place without intense unlearning and trauma work? We don't. We've passed from generation to generation the deeply ingrained sense of captivity that our ancestors felt when they were bound in chains on slave ships crossing the Atlantic, the sense of being free but not yet free that our parents' generation felt during Jim Crow, and the hopelessness we continue to

---

1   "Trauma-Informed Care," Missouri's Early Care & Education Connections, March 4, 2024, https://earlyconnections.mo.gov/professionals/trauma-informed-care; "Trauma," Center for Addiction and Mental Health, www.camh.ca/en/health-info /mental-illness-and-addiction-index/trauma.

witness with the state of institutionalization (private prisons) and other forms of modern-day captivity in our community.

So, before we dive into this work, practice giving yourself compassion as you "wake up" and unlearn. Not only has our society implemented systems to keep you from leaning in to your body's innate wisdom, but it has gaslighted our community into believing the effects of this trauma don't even exist. (As I write this book, I'm reflecting on how I've seen the rolling back of protections of our freedoms as Black people and the banning of books that share details of our history—Black history—in order to hide the atrocities of slavery and present a one-sided view of American history in school textbooks.)

Know that this work is revolutionary. Understanding and exercising ownership of your own body is a form of activism. And in healing yourself, you're disrupting the system that would continue to profit from you not doing so.

Fostering Bodily Awareness

"How does it feel in your body?" This is a question that seems simple but actually is so complex for many of us. When we're accustomed to operating with high cortisol levels in fight-or-flight mode, whether at work or in our homes, it is revolutionary to be able to recognize and honor what we're feeling. Once someone is able to unearth their emotions and how that translates into what they physically feel in their body, the discoveries are profound yet heartbreaking to witness. Heartbreaking because the level of disconnect in Black women is far more than what I've seen facilitating similar spaces for non-Black and nonfemale bodies. This phenomenon is unsurprising, given the high percentage of Black women dealing with diseases and health issues that have been linked to the suppression of emotions and chronic stress, including autoimmune disorders and heart conditions.[2]

Given these realities, the most liberating thing a Black woman can do is have awareness of her own body, to become so in tune with it that she no longer puts off investigating physical discomforts, dis-ease, and most importantly, her own emotions and feelings. After years, even decades, of suppression and neglect, how do you get to that place? You can start by creating consistent, small habits of checking in with yourself throughout the day.

The following prompts will help you begin to create daily habits to reconnect with your body. These are tried-and-true techniques that we've used in our work with beginners (and further highlighted in the "go-deeper exercises" in this book).

- Check in with your breathing. Is it short and shallow, so that your inhales and exhales can only be felt from your collarbone up? Does your chest feel tight? Is your jaw clenched or forehead furrowed? When you notice this tension in your body, can you start by just slowing down your natural breathing, becoming more intentional, and if you're able, elongating those natural inhales and exhales and noticing how your body feels?

---

2   Maytal Eyal, "Self-Silencing Is Making Women Sick," *Time*, October 3, 2023, https://time.com/6319549/silencing-women-sick-essay.

- Use your senses to bring your mind to the present moment and what's accessible to you. Sight: What do you see in the space around you? Smell: What do you smell in the environment you're in? Touch: What surface is supporting you, holding you up in this moment? Hearing: What sounds do your ears pick up on and gravitate to? Allow yourself to sink deeper into that support, affirming you are right where you need to be in this moment.
- Perform a short body scan where you check in with each body part and gauge how it's feeling. Start at the top of your head, moving to your neck, shoulders, chest, stomach, hips, and limbs. Observe any sensations and/or tensions. The goal here is to create a habit of checking in with your body.
- Use your phone to set a few reminders during the day to take a pause in order to check in with yourself, your body, and your energy levels.

Addressing Trauma in the Body

"Breathe in, breathe out" seems like a simple instruction, but as you become one with the breath, you realize the implications of being able to slow down enough to get out of fight-or-flight mode. It is revolutionary to slow down and detach yourself from society's messaging that you're not good enough and will never have enough. It is revolutionary to connect to your body because we didn't always own our bodies, and we couldn't always feed ourselves when we felt hungry. It is revolutionary to slow down enough to turn inward and begin to unpack all the ways in which we've housed trauma—the trauma that we've experienced directly and the trauma that was passed down to us. And it can all start with your breath. Continuous connection with your breath can get you to the point at which you notice where the inhale ends and the exhale begins, you slow down a racing heartbeat, you activate your vagus nerve, and you cultivate more margin around your thoughts. While worries and uncertainties are still present, those thoughts no longer feel as claustrophobic.

CULTIVATING A LOVING RELATIONSHIP WITH YOUR BODY AFTER EXPERIENCING TRAUMA

Recall the example at the beginning of this chapter of experiencing a physical wound and needing the proper care to heal. Similarly, our bodies need a safe space to heal after experiencing a traumatic event. The effects of trauma can show up as a fried nervous system, imbalanced hormones that cause weight gain and menstrual cycle irregularities, and racing, ruminating thoughts and flashbacks. It is not easy to create a space for our bodies to ease into rest in our capitalistic society, but it is so important to do our best to seek a safe haven after traumatic events—whether they occurred yesterday or twenty years ago and are being triggered anew. You may not have a lot of resources or time, given all of your responsibilities, but there are practical, accessible tools you can use in your day-to-day life that can make a difference in the aftermath of trauma.

NURTURING YOUR PHYSICAL BODY

The bodies of Black women have always been under scrutiny. Many of us have not seen skin tones and body types like ours celebrated, and not just sexualized, in mainstream media. So, in addition to nurturing your physical body in the aftermath of a traumatic event, continuously affirm your body to build your self-worth and create a home you'll feel comfortable returning to.

I've seen many community members who have had dysfunctional relationships with their bodies. Whether they'd experienced sexual trauma or were coping with various eating disorders, the disconnection from their bodies ran deep. This detachment can make it even more difficult to provide the tender, loving care that our bodies crave and need after experiencing trauma. There are gentle, compassionate ways for you to connect to your body without an expensive vacation (though you deserve one of those, too, sis) by utilizing everyday routines and rituals to begin relating to your body in a positive way. As we, Black women, experience harm out in the world, we deserve to cultivate a safe home within ourselves.

INDULGING IN REST OF ALL KINDS

After the body has experienced a traumatic event, one of the best prescriptions is to rest. And though partaking in rest after experiencing anything that has taxed our brains and bodies should be a given, as alluded to earlier, it is particularly hard for us Black women. The discomfort felt when many of us find ourselves on an evening with nothing to do and actually have the time and space to pour back into ourselves lets us know that for us to truly engage in rest without guilt or shame, we must practice it. When we usually hear the word *rest*, sleep may be the first thing that comes to mind, but there are many ways for us to engage in practices that help us restore our bodies and minds.

Finding yourself on the other side of processing a specific traumatic event or uncovering long-held, buried traumas can leave you with unending, spiraling thoughts that can be tempting to keep ruminating on, pushing you into a negative headspace. Engaging in mental rest is the medicine needed to find a sense of calm. Activities for mental rest include what I refer to as healthy distractions: allowing yourself to binge-watch your favorite sitcom for an entire weekend, getting lost in someone else's life through a book, or tuning in to a tasteless reality TV show. These types of mental rest provide a mental escape and can have a positive impact in the long run on your healing journey, as they provide a momentary opportunity to "check out" of the heaviness of the situation you're processing.

When it comes to physical rest and allowing yourself to truly, in the words of NaJe, "go lay down," it's normal to feel restless when you finally have the opportunity to do so. Listening to your body's cues for physical rest outside of your nighttime sleep and actually honoring them can be achieved by easing yourself into a practice of doing nothing. If guilt and shame arise for you when you go to take a nap or just want to relax in bed, support your senses by turning on a soothing playlist, burning your favorite candle that evokes a feeling of calm and ease, and putting on your favorite loungewear or pajamas. Help your body feel comfortable and practice listening to its signals that it could use a slowdown with those supportive elements until you find yourself more comfortable taking those breaks sans guilt. And maybe initially you start practicing in five-, ten-, or fifteen-minute intervals until your innate ability to allow yourself to restore your body and nervous system becomes second nature with little internal resistance.

And for your nighttime rest, treat yourself like you would care for a baby. Create a sleep schedule that you adhere to for at least 80 percent of the week. Cultivate an environment that signals and further helps cultivate your mind's association with rest. Designate the couch for watching TV and eating, reading, or working from home. Designate your room as the no–cell phone zone or the place you refuse to take your laptop.

We touch more on hobbies and their importance in exploring our self-identity in chapter 4, but creative rest is also a type of rest that is beneficial to the body as it heals from trauma. Examples of creative rest include activities that can allow you to be expressive and activate the right side of your brain, like painting (or painting-by-numbers if becoming the next Kara Walker is not your goal), knitting, doing puzzles, taking a DJing class, etc.

CLEANSING AND AFFIRMING YOUR BODY

Whether you opt for a shower or a bath, water is restorative. Lather your soap and use a soft washcloth (this is black girls breathing,® after all—if you know, you know). While washing up, express appreciation for every part of your body, especially the parts you feel insecure about or think are flawed or scarred by a difficult life experience. You can even get specific with your gratitude by saying something like "Thank you, hands, for helping me serve myself and others today." Or, "Thank you, legs, for supporting me and allowing me to get from one place to the next today." The list goes on and on. The goal of this practice is to reinforce compassionate, kind, and positive talk about your body to counteract any criticism you may project onto yourself or experience out in the world each day.

NURTURING SELF-TOUCH

Whenever the topic of loneliness surfaced within our community, it was often related to a lack of physical touch and intimacy with a romantic partner. But feeling physically loved and comforted doesn't have to happen solely in the context of romantic relationships or relationships in general. In fact, we can be better partners who are fully open to intimate connection when we have healthy perceptions of our own touch. And please note that I'm not suggesting self-touch is a replacement or filler for romantic love but an opportunity to explore the effects of our own consistent embrace.

When you were a baby, your caregiver(s) gently rocked you to sleep. The back-and-forth motion while being cradled creates a sense of safety for the baby. Though we have grown older, an embrace in a cradled position can still create the same sense of safety in our bodies as adults. Try this out by sitting on the floor with your knees bent and your arms wrapped around your knees.

Gently rock forward and backward with your eyes closed. Keep rocking and allowing your body to sink into this motion for as long as you need to work through any difficult emotions like abandonment or grief that surface. If this practice is not accessible to you, try lying on your side in a curled C position with your arms wrapped around yourself. Massage your arms with your hands, becoming acquainted with the feel of your own touch and embrace.

MIRROR WORK

Growing up taking ballet and pointe classes and being in competitive dance, I was hyperfocused on how my body rarely looked like anyone else's in my classes as a child—so much so that I would purposefully avoid looking at myself in the mirror in class and in front of others. It didn't feel safe in those environments to observe myself fully in that way. As an adult, I got better acquainted with how I looked in the mirror each day. Learning to affirm my reflection no matter what was looking back at me took work. Becoming more comfortable looking at myself allowed me to show up in the world more boldly. I had already seen me, so I was more open to allowing the world to see me, too. Seeing and affirming your body will strengthen your relationship to it and foster greater acceptance that extends to the world around you.

If you've struggled with enjoying what you see in the mirror, carve out an evening when you're winding down and have engaged in a few self-care rituals. When you feel relaxed, sit (if possible) or stand in front of your mirror and simply observe what you see from your head to your toes. Is there anything that you automatically like about your body and what you see? As you examine each part of your body, is there an area that elicits a sense of shame, disgust, or dislike? What words of compassion can you utter to that body part to create more self-acceptance? If you feel moved to make a change beyond awareness, what actions can you take to improve what you do not like seeing? (While you work toward that change, it's important that you continuously affirm your present reality.)

Navigating life after trauma can often make one feel as if they are existing outside of their body. Tools like breathwork help you to tap in to your body and sit with the emotions that arise in spite of the discomfort. For someone who is newly adopting these tools, and even for those of us who have been using them for a long time, the effect can be different and can trigger new sensations and revelations each time. Becoming more in tune with our bodies will help heal our traumas and provide more opportunities to lean in to our body's experience rather than succumbing to avoidance as we explore any unaddressed traumas and different chapters of life.

RECONCILING WITH PAST VERSIONS OF OURSELVES

After we commence deep body work, it may leave us with grief to walk through. Grieving past versions of ourselves who thought so little of ourselves and allowed ourselves to be mistreated over and over again can be a difficult task. For some of us, as we begin to heal, it can be painful to grasp the reality that we were accustomed to permitting partners to feed us only breadcrumbs while we gave our all to the relationship.

The newfound, aware self will have to sift through past versions of itself with compassion and refrain from using today's knowledge to punish the ignorance of yesterday. This practice takes time and consistent rewiring of harmful, spiraling thoughts and self-punishment. How can you see past versions of yourself through the lens of compassion? She didn't know, sis. She didn't know. She was only working with the tools that were passed down or modeled to her, if any at all.

Take a brief moment to close your eyes and envision your former self. Feel her fears and meditate on her beliefs, her perspective of the world, and all that she thought was possible at that time. Sit with her. Cry with her. It's okay to feel sad for her, to grieve all that she missed out on in life because of the tools that were or weren't handed to her. Give her a warm embrace and caress the top of her head like you would a small child. Speaking to her in the same tone that you would use with a dear friend, assure her that she is safe now. She can drop her defenses. You've got her covered and can take this life thing from here. You see her. Show up for her and do the internal work to be the person she needed in her life when she was younger. You are her hero. There is no need for her to search aimlessly for that kind of love to fill the void now. She is that love and that abundant joy. It is innate within her. It always has been there—she's just reawakening to that discovery now.

Take some time to write a letter to that version of you. Give her the encouragement, compassion, and affirmation she needed at that time. What promise will the new you make when it comes to recognizing and tending to her needs moving forward?

Though trauma may have impacted how you've shown up in the world in the past, it doesn't have to continue to do so. We can use the innate wisdom and systems of our bodies to address these long-held traumas and find a sense of freedom, relief, and safety within ourselves first, and hopefully out in the world in the future. I know our ancestors, who did not have autonomy over their own bodies, envisioned a place in the afterlife where all their burdens would be laid down, their problems solved, and their suffering ended. And sis, as you make your way through this deep and— I won't lie to you—sometimes hard work of healing, my greatest wish for you is that you'll find peace within that will trickle into your external world. I wish you peace, sis. You deserve it.

GO-DEEPER EXERCISE: OCEANIC BREATHWORK FOR HEALING THE BODY FROM TRAUMA

This breathwork exercise can be done daily alongside affirmations to rebuild self-trust and self-love after traumatic events. Breathwork is an active form of meditation. It's a great tool for regulating the nervous system and addressing the trauma held in your body and the triggers attached to that trauma; and the oceanic breathwork pattern in particular is great for those who are new to breathwork. (Note: Increasing the amount of oxygen in your brain and blood can make you feel dizzy or lightheaded. This is a normal experience while participating in breathwork, so allow your body to lean in to a new practice that may initially feel uncomfortable while also listening to your body to take breaks when you may need them. It is important to consult a physician before beginning new practices that can have physiological effects.)

The name *oceanic breath* comes from the sound of this practice. For this particular exercise, your mouth is going to be wide-open for increased airflow.

1. Inhale through the mouth, filling your lungs to capacity. Feel your chest rise.
2. Exhale out of the mouth, depleting your lungs. Feel your belly hugging your rib cage.
3. Connect your inhales and exhales in a continuous loop. The inhale imitates waves coming to shore. The exhale sounds like the waves going back out to sea.

Your goal is to tap in to your body with each breath. Focus not on achieving a certain count for inhales and exhales, as we all have different lung capacities (this is a part of my philosophy on why I do not teach any breathwork methodologies that have counts in my work). As you breathe, allow yourself to picture any memories that come to mind of when you felt betrayed, not seen, or unimportant. As those memories surface, gently affirm yourself with each inhale.

Here are some affirmations to guide you through this exercise:

- *I am enough. I am worthy. I will heal my bloodline. I deserve good things. I deserve to give myself rest.*

- *I am not the bad things that have happened to me or my family.*
- *I get to define who I am in this space and time.*
- *I offer grace and healing energy to the pain and suffering experienced in my bloodline.*
- *I offer grace and healing energy to the pain I've experienced myself.*
- *I offer compassion to the little girl within me who did not experience the love or care she needed. I vow to offer that to her now.*
- *I can be who I need to be for myself...right here and right now.*
- *I love who I am and give myself permission to get to know more of who I am.*
- *I find freedom by choosing to be in spaces that honor me.*

Repeat this exercise as long as you need in order to center yourself in the present moment, allowing yourself to create a sense of safety in your body.

Chapter 3

YOUR MAMA, HER MAMA, AND HER MAMA'S MAMA

MY GRANDMOTHER WAS a sharecropper in a small town called Money, Mississippi. You've probably heard of it. It's the same racist town where Emmett Till was brutally murdered in 1955. Central to my grandmother's life was continuous fear and the need to survive. Productivity wasn't just a factor that defined her self-worth, as our capitalistic society teaches us today. No, her productivity was a matter of life or death. It was a daily fight to avoid unwanted sexual encounters, to ensure she produced one hundred–plus pounds of cotton each day for fear of getting beaten, and to help take care of her siblings after her parents died. When she fled for Chicago at age fifteen, it was with the belief that however her life would be in a big city where she knew only her siblings who'd migrated there years before, it couldn't be worse than what her life had been in Mississippi.

I know the harrowing realities of my personal lineage aren't so different from those of other descendants of the African diaspora. For generations, we have had to operate in fight-or-flight mode just to survive. There was constant fear and uncertainty about whether our ancestors would be separated or displaced from their families, become a victim of a random white person's false narrative, or have enough food or a safe shelter to survive. Our ancestors' only objectives were to survive and, if they could, to lessen the pain and suffering experienced by their children. There was no space or time for them to heal or even to begin to understand the psychological, emotional, and physical damage that living in constant fear had caused. They didn't have the space to reflect much on the state of their existence except to strategize the best ways to see another day in spite of all the obstacles.

I've sat at the feet of my maternal grandmother listening to her tell me about her life growing up more times than I can count. But it wasn't until I started focusing on helping Black women heal that I truly began to reflect on all of the ways I'd been personally impacted by the harms committed against my predecessors. There were traumas stored in the cells of my body even though I had not personally gone through those things. These remembrances, perceived and actual limitations, fears, and deep pain that were part of my parents' and grandparents' struggles were now a part of my own healing work.

The trauma experienced by American Black folk (and other members of the African diaspora and victims of colonization) is generational. When we look at our colloquialisms, cultural traditions that are unique to us, and shared experiences that date back to slavery, we see evidence of how we continue to pass down knowledge and inherent ways of being. But along with our joy and ethnic celebrations and contributions to this world, we've also inherited the impact of the violence, separation, and discrimination that our ancestors had to endure. It can feel unfair to know that so many of the limiting beliefs and thought patterns we've had to address came through no fault of our own. But to fully heal, we can't turn a blind eye to the impact of the trauma passed down to us through our bloodline and, for Black women in particular, the trauma we inherited from our maternal figures.

If you were to ask your parents or grandparents what trauma work they've done to process their experience, you probably wouldn't get much of a response. So not only have our bloodlines faced significant horrors, but they have never processed those atrocities and are likely using avoidance, the only tool that was available to them at the time, as a coping mechanism to power through. Now that we live in an age when there is so much information at our fingertips, it's truly a privilege to learn about how our environments and personal histories have impacted us and to be able to adopt tools that can help us heal.

Generational trauma is trauma that gets passed down from one descendant to the next. In our collective histories, we share the impact of trauma caused by cultural, familial, and individual catastrophic events. Think about the fact that American chattel slavery lasted more than two hundred years, and upon formal emancipation, freedom still wasn't fully realized. Our ancestors shifted from enslaved people to supposedly free people who were operating within societal structures that continued to uphold inequality and oppression. From indentured servants to slaves to sharecroppers, our lineage experienced modified forms of enslavement over time. Their labor was worth mere pennies that then had to be paid against imaginary and ever-changing debts imposed by plantation owners, maintaining systems of inequity. The impact of these centuries-long traumas still hasn't received proper acknowledgment or recompense on a national or individual level (I would even suggest that many Americans respond to our traumas with gaslighting). The result is that we are still working to get free of invisible chains today so that we can be seen as equals and feel respected, honored, and valued in the world.

An experience as traumatic and prolonged as slavery impacts our very brain chemistry and the expression of our DNA, a phenomenon studied in the field of epigenetics. While we can't change some characteristics that are passed down to us, like hair and eye color, body shape, and facial features, we aren't doomed to suffer the effects of trauma for the rest of our lives. Addressing instead of suppressing the realities of this painful trauma will require walking through anger, extreme sadness, and hopelessness, but we can get to the other side thanks to our ancestors who fought for us to survive and thrive.

THE WEIGHT OF GENERATIONAL TRAUMA

The emotional and mental energy required to sort through not just our own stuff but also the traumas of our ancestors is immense. And that's why addressing mental and emotional health is so complex for us Black women. We house the traumas of being Black in a racist world, as well as the traumas of being women in a sexist world, in our bodies.

We carry the weight of often needing to be the backbone

of our families in a country that lacks adequate social resources for our community. We are the safety nets in our families and communities because no one else is stepping in. The effects of slavery and oppression on Black people—and on Black women in particular—continue to ripple from generation to generation, compounding as the trauma remains unaddressed and unhealed. While we are no longer bound by physical shackles, oppression has shape-shifted into invisible chains, ranging from mass incarceration impacting Black men and Black families to extreme wealth inequality that has only gotten worse over time. In this world, we are far from free. To change that, we must start by going deep into the body.

For us Black women who have dared to do the arduous work of unlearning destructive patterns and to heal from the traumas getting in the way of living a more fulfilling life, we may hit an impasse once we recognize the depth of our traumas and where they originated. We may feel overwhelmed by despair when we consider the multiple generations of trauma that preceded us and continue to affect us, as well as righteous anger over the injustices that created this trauma.

GRIEVING THE CHILDHOOD YOU NEVER HAD

When you dig deeper into your childhood, you may observe beliefs, behavioral patterns, and ways of being that were passed down to you but that you want to rewrite now that you're an adult. Sometimes, it wasn't just what was said and done that had a big impact on your psyche, but also what was left unsaid and undone.

Children crave order, affection, and affirmation. Many Black women experienced harsh childhoods in which we did not receive a lot of affection or feel seen or welcome to fully express our emotions, thoughts, and opinions. We understand that our elders often lacked the parental tools to function outside of survival mode, but when this leaves us feeling unprepared to thrive in the world as adults, we often feel cheated, not only by systemic injustices but by how these injustices in the outside world leaked into what was supposed to be our safest space. And if one decides to let their parents in on this realization, they often end up getting defensive, as it was nearly impossible to provide a healthy, affirming childhood when they were barely making it, often as the first in their family to attain a certain level of education or enter their profession. How could they have had the emotional capacity to provide more than they actually had, given all that they were carrying and the fact that therapy and other healing modalities just weren't something Black folks did back then? From their perspective, they did more than enough in light of the reality they were forced to navigate and their experience being raised by their own parents. We cannot blame them for doing the best they could with what they had. To suggest otherwise might be seen as a lack of appreciation and respect for all of their sacrifices. An important part of the unlearning phase is to affirm your own truths. Seek deeper understanding and solace for your own healing by creating emotional distance from your parents' response, acknowledging your different perspectives, and offering them forgiveness and understanding that they truly may have done the best they could with the tools they had.

As a result of our parents' hypervigilance to keep us safe, the message that many of us received in childhood was to stay small and avoid rocking the boat in any way, shape, or form. "Only speak when spoken to." "Stay out of grown folks' business." "I'm only harsh to you because I love you." As a result of generational trauma, many of us rarely experienced affirming, gentle, yet corrective love in our childhoods. Instead, we were taught in childhood to be prepped for battle and obstacles in the outside world and to strive for perfection and excellence. We are left to grapple with the fact that our innocence was stolen from us at an early age. What would our childhoods have looked like if our parents', grandparents', great-grandparents', and great-great-grandparents' lives weren't hijacked by oppression and violence? How would they have been able to model self-care, self-love, and living out their dreams if they'd been allowed to live freely, without constantly needing to defend themselves or react to real and potential dangers around them? Perhaps you've envisioned what that reality would have looked like. Although we deserve to give voice to our anger over all that has been lost and stolen from us, we must also do the healing work to limit the traumas passed on to the next generation so that we can reclaim our collective and individual power. We can't erase the pain our lineage endured. And even though we are still experiencing the injustices of this world to some degree, I have to believe that we have the opportunity to represent a major turning point in our bloodlines. We can choose to be heroes for our younger selves and future generations, a privilege our ancestors dreamed to give us, in spite of the inadvertent harm that was passed down as a result of their need to survive.

SELF-DEPRECATION AS A COPING MECHANISM

One aspect of the generational trauma that I often see Black women needing to address is the effects of our maternal figures' tendency to put us down, an instinct that originated in their desire to protect us. Our maternal ancestors who were enslaved would try to keep their daughters safe from the master's lustful urges or from getting sold off to another plantation by regularly demeaning their daughters in his presence. "She's not anything." "She ain't that pretty." "She won't be nothing." Obviously, these were different times and conditions than the world we live in, where most parents are trying to raise emotionally whole and confident children. But under those circumstances—stripped of previous cultures and family structures (families were often broken up and sold to different owners)—those were the only tools that our ancestors had to survive.

What does this mean for the Black women who join our black girls breathing® community to heal their mother wounds? Some of the tools that were used to keep daughters safe while in captivity are still being used to some extent in the present day. Our bodies still house the traumas experienced on the fields and during Jim Crow, even though the threats we experience today aren't the same as the threats experienced under enslavement. Black girls today are indirectly taught to be self-deprecating, and they end up growing into Black women who lack self-esteem and the sense of security and self-worth they need to navigate the world. Until one Black girl turned woman in that lineage decides to do the deeper work to understand the whys behind her family's behavior, the cycle will, unfortunately, continue. Black girls deserve to feel beautiful and to be complimented. Black girls deserve to affirm and big-up themselves without fearing that they'll be accused of their head "getting too big." What would it look like for Black girls to first see their potential and receive affirmation of their brilliance and beauty from their moms? What would it look like if our mothers had the capacity, tools, and freedom to show up as a nurturer first, rather than a fearful protector due to their own experiences in the world that hardened them? In recognizing the rough edges of our mothers' and other maternal figures' love, we understand that they're doing the best they can with the tools they were given to protect their daughters and help them survive. But now we recognize that it is safe enough in our bodies and our homes to adopt new tools.

THE DIFFERENCES IN RAISING GIRLS VERSUS BOYS

I've heard many Black women who grew up with at least one brother recount how they had to deal with issues that their brothers never had to deal with. Oftentimes, girls are overprepared for the real world while boys are coddled. Girls aren't just taught the basics of cooking, cleaning, and doing laundry; they must master these tasks, often even performing these responsibilities for their brothers.

As a result, girls absorb the message that men are to be catered to. It's assumed that boys aren't organized enough to perform similar duties, no matter their age. Girls are expected to grow up and mature faster than boys, to trade in their childhood for more responsibilities that their mothers can no longer handle on their own. Girls rarely, if ever, see their fathers chip in. Rather than ask her male partner for help, a mother shifts responsibility to her daughter.

Early on, Black girls are carrying responsibilities and worries that are much too mature and heavy for their age. They are concerned about their households running smoothy, not just in terms of chores, but making sure that everyone's moods are stable, on top of the other duties on their plates, like school and extracurriculars. Girls are taught at an early age to get used to carrying heavy loads with grace and without complaint. At the same time, they are taught to not hold their male counterparts to the same standard. Girls are taught to see boys as not as capable and to protect their boyhood and freedom by taking as much worry and responsibility off their plates as possible, given the heavy loads that these boys have to carry out in the world. Girls are told "Boys will be boys" and "Well, you're not a boy so you can't do that." This familiar rhetoric follows them as they transition from girlhood to teenager to young adult. Girls will temper their exploration, growth, and curiosity in response to others' fears. Girls don't want to be seen as "fast," unlovable, or unworthy. The impact of this conditioning creates work for our adult selves to explore with our inner child.

ACKNOWLEDGING YOUR INNER CHILD

Have you ever been in a grocery store and seen a child throwing a tantrum, yelling, and screaming? It may have come out of nowhere and embarrassed the caregiver, who may have apologetically told passersby, "They're usually well-behaved" or "They don't usually act like this." Similarly, our inner child can show up suddenly in our lives when we have been ignoring the layers of unaddressed trauma in our bodies. Our inner child will try to communicate their wounds to us if they haven't received adequate attention. Our inner child might not feel prioritized or safe to explore emotions that our adult selves would rather suppress and ignore. This coping strategy often gets reinforced in our capitalistic society, where we have little time to rest, grieve (often with a one- to two-day bereavement period), or even focus our attention on ourselves when there is constant distraction from our phones and social media.

In my own journey and the journeys of others, I've seen the inner child appear when we do not feel at home in our bodies, when we are disconnected from our emotions, and when physical symptoms such as aches and pains emerge. Failing to acknowledge the deep wounds of childhood and the truths that our inner child is anxiously waiting to reveal to us can indeed cause symptoms in our bodies. This can manifest in what could be described as an adult tantrum: the inability to regulate our emotions, feeling agitated, and experiencing depressive bouts and high levels of anxiety.

Our inner child can't analyze our emotions and wounds in the same way that the adult mind can. The inner child often sees the world through the same lens and with the same level of emotional maturity as when the trauma or wound first happened. Given the lack of mental and emotional resources available to our families and communities, those wounds likely went unacknowledged by our caregivers. If your family experienced generational traumas, returning to the wounds of your younger years may be the medicine you need to heal. Our younger selves couldn't mentally process everything they experienced, and we've now come to realize in adulthood that our parents and their parents did their best with the tools that were available to them. This understanding allows us to stop internalizing our parents' actions the way we did when we were younger, when we interpreted their disapproval and lack of attention or affirmation as abandonment or something being wrong with us.

LEARNING TO SPEAK UP AFTER BEING SILENCED

If generational trauma has caused you to suppress your emotions or resort to other coping mechanisms, it's likely that your inner child is longing to express herself and be heard. Think of our ancestors who lived and worked on plantations. So much of their existence was erased. They avoided drawing attention to themselves and did not want to be seen or heard in order to protect themselves; they focused on the work of their hands. They had to tend to the crops, cook food and have it ready on the table, and listen intently for anyone requesting their presence or making a demand without being able to socialize or spend much time with their kin, except maybe on Sundays. How do you think this history influenced what was taught, whether explicitly or implicitly, from generation to generation? Long after we had left the fields, we continued to experience a fear of vocalizing our emotions, needs, and wants. And how does this affect us today?

I've met so many Black women who have a deep fear of self-expression. Being able to acknowledge what they want, how they're feeling, and their hopes and dreams takes practice after many generations of having their voice (and identity) suppressed. Since we were told as young children to open our mouths only when spoken to, we've grown into adults who struggle with speaking up. How can you now give yourself permission to speak and express yourself more freely? How do you begin to feel comfortable enough to do more than just appease others, as you were conditioned to do as a child with your overtaxed parents? We'll explore many tools for finding and cultivating our sense of self throughout this book, but we must first take stock of how we may have been silenced during our childhood so we can directly address it and heal.

HEALING YOUR MOTHER WOUND

Our bonds with our mothers and maternal figures specifically shape so much of how we view ourselves, define womanhood and motherhood, and navigate relationships with other women, both subconsciously and consciously. A mother who was exhausted from work and/or domestic duties at home while also caring for her children most likely didn't have the capacity to invest more than the bare minimum to keep her children fed, clothed, and on time for school. And though she was doing her best, her lack of attention and maybe even her expectation that you take on some of the adult household responsibilities likely had an effect on you. When you think about your relationship with your mother or mother figure growing up, what emotions immediately come up for you? Maybe they're resentment or pain. Maybe they're deep compassion and sadness as you reflect on her struggles, which you were unable to recognize as a child but are more apparent to you now as an adult. Even as we extend compassion to our maternal caregivers, we also validate our need for their nurture and recognize the very real pain of our inner child. Once we acknowledge this need that went unmet, we can take a deeper look at how the wound formed in the first place.

Many core wounds begin in childhood, perhaps because of a traumatic event or ongoing exposure to a stressful environment. When you reflect on your childhood, are there any specific instances you recall of seeking your mother's approval, affection, or attention but not receiving it? How did that make you feel?

WHAT YOU LEARNED FROM YOUR MOTHER

Let's take the opportunity to explore any beliefs that you absorbed during your childhood that stem from your relationship with your mother. Take a few minutes to complete this exercise and honor whatever response first comes up for you in your body and mind.

Choose among the following in response to each prompt—keep in mind that our beliefs are based on not always facts but how we feel and how our inner child has interpreted a situation:

ALWAYS | MOST TIMES | SOMETIMES | RARELY | NEVER

1. I knew my mom / maternal figure loved me from her actions and how she made me feel growing up.

2. I saw my mom / maternal figure regularly make time for herself and prioritize her needs. She taught me how to care for myself and prioritize obligations accordingly.

3. I saw my mom / maternal figure receive love from her mom, even as an adult.

4. I felt my mom / maternal figure was active and present in my life and cared about my interests growing up.

5. When I was angry, sad, lonely, or disappointed, my mom / maternal figure validated those feelings and allowed me to express them fully.

Observe your immediate response to each prompt. Closing your eyes, picture the younger version of yourself. Reflect on each answer and a specific scenario that gave you that impression of your mother. What emotions are coming up for you? Where are they housed in your body? How can you affirm your younger self's feelings and address those needs now as an adult? How can you let your inner child know that it is safe now and that as an adult, you can provide the nurturing that you need? (Hint: create some affirmations to practice reinforcing these newfound truths to your inner child.)

WHEN YOU'RE READY FOR FORGIVENESS

The most difficult stage of healing parental wounds for many is forgiveness. You may feel righteous anger when you uncover and grieve aspects of your childhood that you missed out on and when you imagine possibilities of who you could be and how your life would be different if you had received more love from your caregivers or if you hadn't experienced or witnessed traumatic events. With the knowledge you have now, you can see the missteps made by your guardians and how you would have done so many things differently. It's important for me to validate this phase of your healing journey, when you might not be ready to forgive right away. It's okay to allow yourself to feel all of the emotions and set appropriate boundaries if you do not have the kind of relationship with your parents where you can talk to them directly about the truths of your childhood. If you can't talk to your parents, it might be helpful to explore some of these hard truths with a trusted older figure. While your adult self might not need it, this can be a productive exercise for your inner child to feel seen, heard, and accepted by a mentor figure. You will be receiving affirmation from someone else while also listening to and validating your own feelings and making space for your inner child to express disappointments. I believe that though it is important to take ownership of our healing, there are ways for us to involve our community in the process, as humans are designed for connection, and not all healing can be done alone.

Taking time to reflect on how you see your parents can be beneficial for your own healing as well. What are the specific scenarios that impacted how they showed up as caregivers? What did they not unlearn from their parents that negatively impacted you and your upbringing? How can you offer compassion to their inner child, who likely didn't have their needs met, while also holding space for your real, lived experience? (I'm definitely not asking you to ignore or avoid your truths in order to offer compassion, sis. I do believe we can hold multiple emotions and truths at the same time.) How has what they learned over their lifetimes prevented them from understanding or taking accountability for the negative impacts of unhealed trauma on how they raised you and your siblings? With that information in mind, how can you begin to make peace with what they were able to provide, and even offer forgiveness (it can be internal and not expressed directly to them) in order for your inner child to experience more peace about aspects of their life's journey that can't be rewritten but can be healed?

Once you've forgiven or at least processed the wounds of your childhood, especially related to your relationship with your mother, you can begin to actively rewire certain beliefs and heal your inner child by providing what your mother couldn't. By addressing the traumas that were caused by parental figures and doing the brave work of healing, you'll relieve yourself of the burden of continuing to carry wounds that did not start, but that will end, with you.

GO-DEEPER EXERCISE: ENVISIONING
ANCESTRAL HEALING

Begin by picturing your mother, grandmother, or other maternal figure in your lineage. Now envision, to the best of your ability, her younger, childlike self. See her innocence and joy. Knowing what you've explored in your lineage and the traumas she's endured, see your adult self gifting her with what her inner child needed. What affirmations would you say to her inner child? How would you express unconditional love to her? What actions could you take to make her feel safe, in spite of all that was happening in her outside world? Now, considering what you know about the traumas she experienced in adulthood, picture yourself offering her forgiveness for any of her actions that impacted you and your childhood. Observe all the emotions that arise while completing this exercise. Take note of how your body feels. Now let's offer ourselves tender nurturing with the breath, as heavy emotions and energy were likely kicked up.

BREATHWORK EXERCISE FOR RELEASING
CHILDHOOD WOUNDS: THREE-PART BREATH
(TWO INHALES, ONE EXHALE)

1. Get settled in a comfortable position to facilitate this exercise (e.g., lying down, sitting on the floor, or whatever feels most comfortable to you).

2. Begin with your mouth wide-open for increased airflow. Inhale into the mouth, halfway filling up your lungs and

breathing into your stomach area. Then inhale into the mouth again, filling up the rest of your lungs and breathing into your chest area. Feel your entire upper body expand.

3. Exhale out of the mouth, until your belly has collapsed completely. Inhale into the mouth twice (focusing on your stomach area, then your chest area); exhale out of the mouth once. Repeat.

4. While doing this exercise, focus on any energy from unaddressed generational trauma that you're ready to release. What feelings, pain, or energy does your bloodline no longer need? What are you calling into your lineage for your descendants to receive? Use the exhale to release what is ready to go and the inhale to call in what you want more of.

5. Allow yourself to experiment with the time duration when you do this exercise. Perhaps for the first time, do fifteen minutes of active breathwork. Then the next time, try twenty minutes.

Chapter 4

A BLACK WOMAN'S CARE

THE SUMMER OF 2020, George Floyd's death sparked an increase in awareness of the Black Lives Matter movement. And the initiatives that sprung up and gained the most momentum had one thing in common: they were being led by Black women. From marching to ensuring people got out to vote at the polls, Black women were at the forefront, driving change for equal rights for us all—but not without the costs of bearing such a heavy load. Yes, we helped turn purple states blue, but we were also receiving a disproportionately high number of negative health diagnoses that could be linked to chronic stress caused by bearing everyone and their mama's loads. We are heralded for our hard labor, especially when it comes to activism and moving the needle forward. But is the progress worth our harm? When do we scale back and slow down, recognizing that this pace is unsustainable and, quite frankly, killing us?

Maybe we're afraid of what the world would look like without our deep empathy. But perhaps it's time to imagine a world where the empathy we extend to others is the same empathy we give to ourselves. When caring for others is so deeply ingrained in our role as Black women, it can be hard to come to terms with the idea that without our care, a foster kid may end up in the wrong home, a homeless man may not eat for the night, or our mother will be in a nursing home. Sometimes we attribute our lack of self-care to just not having enough time to pour into ourselves, but in fact, we may be pouring into others' well-being at the expense of our own. Perhaps it's time to give the world the opportunity to rise to the occasion without our deep, unfettered sacrifices. Maybe we're so used to striving for perfection and being capable of coming to the rescue that to drop that role would make us question our own worth and position in the world. Because if we're not helping or working to push some agenda forward, then what are we doing? Resting? Oh, no, ma'am—we just can't have that. I think we've overidentified with taking care of others as our rightful place. I'm not saying that we should be indifferent to the world around us, but our health and ability to thrive demand that we care a little less, trusting that the world will continue to spin just fine without our self-deprivation.

THE EFFECTS OF SECONDHAND TRAUMA

The beginning of the COVID-19 pandemic introduced a new norm that involved living in isolation, joining virtual communities, and working from home. While the introverts of the world, myself included, reveled in the opportunity to enjoy solitude and quiet time sans guilt, living without community began to wear on us. The need to connect created high demand for black girls breathing® as the pandemic further widened health and economic disparities for Black women. Many of them were first responders who were overtaxed from the wear and tear of working eighteen-hour days on the frontlines with the ever-present worry of witnessing yet another person's life cut short or catching COVID themselves and potentially spreading it to their loved ones. While some industries thrived during the pandemic, economic gaps widened for service and retail workers who no longer had a reliable source of income. There was only so much that $1,400 in economic relief from the government and unemployment benefits (if you qualified) could do. Women in our community took on the equivalent of second or third jobs at home—on top of cooking and cleaning and working their full-time job, they were now also tasked with being the primary caregiver for an elderly relative and/or helping children navigate virtual school. The wear and tear was felt across the board for people of all ages, walks of life, and socioeconomic backgrounds.

Secondhand trauma is also known as compassion fatigue because it's a form of distress caused by witnessing the aftermath or hearing the details of trauma experienced by other people.[1]

---

1   "Secondary Trauma: Signs, Symptoms, & Treatment," Banyan Treatment Centers, accessed March 15, 2024, www.banyanmentalhealth.com/2022/03/02/secondary -trauma-symptoms.

While making space for these women in our black girls breathing® sessions, I witnessed the erosion of their sanity, and the effects of their traumas began to have a ripple effect on me. This exemplified how we as Black women often take on the worries of those in close proximity to us, mostly due to hundreds of years of conditioning. Our work at black girls breathing® exponentially grew in the span of a month while we simultaneously switched our business model to be more accessible because we noticed how limited financial resources were affecting many long-term members' ability to continue to participate. Recognizing the need, I launched a crowdfunding campaign to provide a year's worth of free breathwork sessions for those in our community who lacked the financial resources to help manage their mental health. What used to be a live group of 25 turned into live groups of 150 to 200; others viewed the recording after the session, with a total of 450 to 500 sign-ups per session.

The world's awareness of the Black Lives Matter movement remained top of mind as we witnessed one Black body after another fall to police violence, deprived of any decency as their last breaths became viral moments. The heaviness of the burdens borne by our community was beyond belief. Though I did my best to leave the weight of each session in the session, it would take days for me to process the traumatic stories that people shared with me. I saw myself and the women in my family in these women's stories, which differed from what I saw in the corporate sessions that were also being booked frequently at that time as employers sought to offer mental health support for employees working through collective grief and isolation. It was harder for me to step away and dissociate from the narratives I heard in our black girls breathing® community. And like many of these women carrying the extra weight of other people's trauma, I began to feel a depressive cloud hanging over me because of the constant exposure to others' real and deep pain. I believe that experiencing this secondhand trauma triggered the development of a health condition that I'm still navigating today.

Despite my work encouraging Black women to take care of themselves, it took me a while to slow down for the same reason that many Black women overtax themselves: other people need us. The women in our black girls breathing® community kept telling me that they needed these sessions to get through their week, so despite my burnout, I asked myself, *If I don't continue, where will they go?* This question often leads to a level of burnout that is way too familiar to Black women.

As many of us have a tendency to do, I rationalized continuing to take on this heavy workload, even as I began to experience physical symptoms like unexplainable fatigue. I attributed the fatigue to the long hours I was working, and given the persistent and all-too-familiar dismissal by my doctor, who said that nothing was wrong, I pressed on with the status quo, including my usual self-care routines: therapy, working out and long walks, breathwork, and quiet time. I realized too late that what had sufficed in previous seasons of my life was no longer enough, given my heightened level of stress. As I write this, I'm now navigating an autoimmune condition that hasn't previously occurred in my family's history. I firmly believe that my exposure to so much trauma during that time is the culprit of this condition. Symptoms worsened over the course of three years before I finally found a primary care provider who agreed to do additional testing. Unsurprisingly, it was a Black woman specialist doctor who took my symptoms seriously and therefore asked me one question that planted the seed in my mind to ask my primary physician for that form of testing.

I hope my story further illustrates my point here, sis: chronic stress is affecting us. I'm not an exception. The consequences of not slowing down snuck up on me and contributed to my decision to finally share this story courageously and vulnerably. I share this warning from a place of love: our rest and our care for ourselves, no matter how inconvenient to others, cannot wait.

RELEASING THE NEED TO SAVE

Although it may be second nature to you to equate your value with how much you do for others, this habit is detrimental in the long term. The moment when life shows up and interrupts your ability to care for others will trigger a sense of identity loss, which might be exacerbated by others' response to your withdrawal of care. Sis, can I ask you something? Who would you be and how would you feel if you tried opting out? If you practiced not being the first in line to come to someone's rescue or defense? And better yet, what do you think it says about you if you're not the epitome of care? Are you selfish? Do you lack compassion for your community?

I often see this dynamic of needing to save, heal, and self-sacrifice when it comes to a lot of Black women's romantic relationships in particular. Women's innate sense of nurture coupled with Black women's social conditioning to be of use leads many to stay in relationships that have "potential" or are downright harmful, to the detriment of the woman. When faced with a partner's indifference or the reality that the relationship is going nowhere, she considers it her duty to try to save the relationship through her actions alone. She takes on full responsibility for the relationship, assuming that her partner will finally see her worth and value her care one day. This is a vicious cycle and a trap created by societal norms and a natural human desire to be seen in a relationship. We shouldn't beat ourselves up if we notice this pattern in our own lives, but seeing the truth gives us an opportunity to choose differently in the future.

In order to break this deeply entrenched pattern, it's important to pause and learn to slow down so we don't automatically default to old, unconscious behavior. In a capitalistic society that teaches us to act fast or we'll miss out, delaying action and resisting a natural urge to rush to someone's rescue without first checking in with ourselves is both countercultural and the first step to deprogramming ourselves from a "care-centered" identity.

THE TWENTY-FOUR-HOUR RULE

When it comes to practicing emotional regulation, taking a pause is a simple yet underrated tool. In order to unlearn deeply ingrained behavior, we need to give ourselves enough time to choose a different behavior over and over again, until we establish a new habit. This practice takes patience and self-compassion. Even when we do all of this internal work, sometimes we find ourselves in situations that trigger old responses and ways of being. When that happens, negative self-talk and shaming ourselves will never get us closer to our goal. Healing isn't a linear path, so focus on progress over perfection.

In order to resist the need to be someone's savior and main source of care, avoid jumping into action at the drop of a hat and honor your present moment's needs. For example, when you get a text message or a phone call with a request (perhaps disguised as a regular check-in, whether it's from a friend, partner, or boss), practice advocating for yourself by not letting the surprise request pressure you into committing to help right away. Prepare yourself for situations like these by thinking about potential responses ahead of time, like "Hmm...let me get back to you on that" or "I'll have to circle back with you later." Choose a response that feels comfortable for you and gives you the space to check in with yourself and assess if you'd like to take on this request or if you'd rather say no (despite the pressure to do otherwise). After you reach a decision, give yourself twenty-four hours to sit with it before responding. This pause is an opportunity not only for you to practice self-advocacy but for those around you to learn a new way of relating to you and your needs.

I don't recommend telling white lies or making up elaborate stories to get out of doing something, because this implies that honoring your needs isn't reason enough. You don't need a long excuse or a fully booked schedule to say no. This practice also strengthens your sense of self and your ability to honor your own needs without external validation. A simple pause can help you to stop responding from a reactive need to be the go-to support person.

During this twenty-four-hour waiting space, observe all the emotions and thoughts that come up for you. Open up the Notes app or audio recorder on your phone or pull out a good ol'-fashioned journal and reflect on how you feel. Are you angry that you even have to practice this exercise? Do you feel upset or manipulated because someone turned what you thought would be a genuine check-in conversation into an opportunity to ask for a favor? These are normal emotions, so allow them to surface fully. There's a lot of stigma around feeling anger, but it's a useful tool to identify all the ways we didn't advocate for ourselves and prioritized others' needs above our own so that it's become difficult for us to even recognize what our needs are. Anger can also indicate that someone's actions toward us simply didn't feel good. This information helps us create better boundaries in the future. And it's okay, sis. Know that it's okay. It takes time to unearth deeply ingrained ways of being. Be proud of yourself for even deciding to do this work at this time. You're not too late to explore all of who you are and unpack other sides of your identity that have nothing to do with how you care for the people around you.

SELF-EXPLORATION THROUGH FUN AND CREATIVE HOBBIES

Many people, Black women chief among them, have a difficult time identifying their needs and preferences—including what they like and don't like and what they're curious about. Since

Black women have been conditioned to prioritize those around us, it can feel awkward or foreign to turn our attention inward. Self-exploration doesn't have to be a daunting task reserved for a therapist's office; it can be as simple and fun as exploring some hobbies.

What have you always wanted to try but never did because you thought you were too old, or you were worried about how you'd be perceived, or you didn't think you had enough time (the excuse I hear most often)? I'd implore you to start there. The curiosity is bursting within you because it has yet to be explored. And healing doesn't have to be so serious all the time, sis. (I personally can't imagine a life where all I do is focus on intensive healing practices.)

I renewed my commitment to explore creative hobbies while writing this book in order to reduce daily stress, especially in light of new health challenges. I wanted some of my new stress relievers to be creative and fun, so I started by reflecting back on my childhood. What used to be fun for me as a child? I used to dance and play the piano and violin—dance and piano were my favorites. I thought about why I'd stopped playing piano and realized that I no longer enjoyed it when an element of competition was introduced. I remember my excitement fading once I began having private lessons with my piano teacher in order to prepare for annual recitals. It was no longer an activity that I could get lost in, just tinkering on the keys and seeing where it led. Piano was now associated with striving for perfection and getting tapped on my knuckles with a pencil whenever I made a mistake. Simply recalling why I'd stopped playing brought up all the negative beliefs I'd internalized that prevented me from exploring that and other hobbies without an end goal in mind. Society taught me as I grew up that there was no room for curiosity and fun for their own sake.

However, making space to foster curiosity will strengthen your ability to try new things without needing to be perfect all the time. It will fortify your self-confidence as you learn new skills and open yourself to exploration without knowing the outcome. There's no pressure to achieve a specific result and, given all the other pressures you experience at work and at home, you need an outlet that is free of any expectation or burden.

My mom's house, where my grandmother also lives since my mom is a full-time caregiver, gave me a sense of nostalgia and was the perfect cocoon to practice the piano and rework those negative beliefs to explore without expectations that I picked up in childhood. I experienced a visceral reaction to sitting on the piano bench that I had to work through, but I was determined to give myself the space to explore playing by ear. It was awkward at first to not have sheet music to guide me but to rely on my ear and allow my fingers to go where they wanted. I reminded myself that there was no one to tap my knuckles when I made a mistake. It was only me and my inner child who wanted to give this a try. I laughed at myself when I hit the wrong notes. I sang aloud as I tried to find the right placement for my fingers, and with time, I was able to play the intro to Q-Tip's "Gettin' Up" by ear. Just witnessing myself figure it out through that process gave me a confidence that translated to other areas of my life and even made me want to explore other hobbies.

Consistently immersing yourself in this kind of creative

process will bear fruits in terms of how you show up in life in general. You'll learn to trust your ability to handle unexpected situations as they come, feel less anxiety about the future, and be able to enjoy life a lot more—all while exploring your interests and different ways of being. As you detach from your identity as a caregiver and begin exploring new identities through hobbies unrelated to achievement, you can further strengthen your sense of self.

CULTIVATING A STRONG SENSE OF SELF

How do you show up for yourself when you're alone in a safe space? How do you integrate the healing work that you've done internally with how you show up in the world with family, friends, and coworkers? People often get discouraged when they try to sustain their healing work amid other people's resistance. It can feel like you've made so much progress centering yourself and your needs, only to question it when you feel triggered by the people around you. Please know that this is part of the journey. I often hear people say, "I've been redefining who I am, so why do I still care so deeply about how others perceive me?" This may feel like regression, but it's actually just an opportunity to keep practicing and applying the tools you've been cultivating.

Remember earlier in this chapter when we talked about allowing ourselves to feel anger when we recognize that we're being used by other people? Let's apply the same technique when we encounter points of friction as we show up in the world in new ways. When we begin to prioritize our own needs, it is common to experience guilt and regret as others respond to the healing work we'd previously only done in isolation. We may be tempted to withdraw or revert to catering to everyone else's needs in order to avoid sitting with the difficult feeling that we've let someone else down. Normalizing this discomfort is part of the growing process as we build the muscles to maintain our boundaries and our new identity amid others' disappointment. Let's explore some examples of old roles that you may want to relinquish.

Scenario: The Primary Caregiver

You take care of most of your elderly parent's needs despite being one of six siblings. You schedule and take your parent to doctors' appointments, cook meals, and bathe and clean up after them on a daily basis, among other duties. After years of keeping up with this routine, you're burned out. The uneven division of labor among your siblings has persisted for far too long. You recognize how your siblings reap the fruit of your tedious labor when they show up only during the holidays to hang with their aging parent or call without any regard to the schedule you maintain for your parent to help you get through the day. You begin to pull back from all the responsibilities, asking specific family members to assist with duties so you can make more time for your own interests and needs. This is met with resistance from your siblings. After all, the pattern has already been established that you are the go-to caregiver, which is highly unsustainable. Although the increased freedom and mental capacity for other things energizes you at first, guilt slowly starts to creep in. You think, *I can't just leave my mom out to hang like that* or *They don't know how to care for her like I do.*

These reactions are to be expected, given how long you've played the role of caregiver, and you'll need to make space for them, allowing your body to feel these emotions. The guilt, regret, and shame you may experience from creating a new identity that isn't based solely on caregiving will be uncomfortable. Pull out your journal, your Notes app, or whatever works for you and document these feelings. Notice how these feelings are rooted in the deeply held belief that your identity and value come from being a caregiver. Even as you validate these emotions, affirm the choice you've made to create a new identity that isn't centered on caregiving. And of course, use the power of breathwork to make a safe space in your body to sit with and feel these feelings. It may take some getting used to, but as with any new practice, you will feel more comfortable sitting with those emotions over time.

Scenario: The Devoted Friend

You pride yourself on being a good friend. When someone in your friend group has a problem, needs advice, or wants to share good news with someone who'll be just as excited as they are, they come to you. Ol' Faithful. Friends may describe you as reliable, someone that they know will always be there for them. Over time, as you do more healing work and go to therapy, you realize that while you like to be dependable, this level of commitment is coming at your expense. Lately, you've been navigating a particularly difficult chapter in life. Although you're normally self-reliant and don't want to burden other people with your problems, you decide that you finally need to lean on someone else for a change. But to your surprise, despite all you've sown into friendships over the years, you find that when you begin reaching out to different friends to let them know you're going through a rough time and could use some support, you don't receive the same energy that you typically give. Some friends don't answer your phone calls or texts. Others simply respond with "I'll get back to you, girl!" And then several weeks go by.

At first, you're upset and wonder, *How could they treat me like this after all the times I've shown up for them?* But then, as time goes by, you realize that you played a part in this relationship dynamic. Since you never asked anything of your friends but always kept a cool head and an "I'll figure it out" attitude, your friends got used to your not needing them. Whether consciously or unconsciously, they started viewing you as the strongest of the group and the friend who always has it all together. In your difficult season, they might think, *She doesn't* really *need me. She'll figure out how to navigate this rough patch on her own, as she always does. Plus, what am I going to say? I don't know how to comfort her as well as she comforts other people. I'm not as strong as her!* That's just one example of how your friends might respond. These situations teach us to be intentional about choosing friends who pour into us as much as we pour into them and to be mindful of how our disposition can create patterns that might be difficult, but not impossible, to reverse in our relationships.

Scenario: The Compassionate Leader

Over the course of your career, you've had some awful managers and traumatic work experiences. So now that you've worked your way to the top, you use every opportunity that you can to create a kinder, more just working environment. You advocate for your direct reports to receive higher pay than average in your industry or company. You encourage them to take on projects that will help them to learn and lead, setting them up for success and growth beyond their current position. You tend to see the good and the potential in every employee.

Over time, you notice one employee who isn't performing like they said they would, and when other colleagues complain about how they're not contributing to the team, you have to have multiple conversations with them to get to the bottom of things. They say they're trying but they're going through various things in their personal life that prevent them from performing at their best. You leave those conversations agreeing to adjust performance metrics just to accommodate them. Coworkers continue to complain. You keep listening and offering grace until you realize that your trust and belief in this person are totally unfounded because you've never seen them consistently produce good, timely work. You only ever saw their potential and bought into their many stories and excuses that produced empathy on your end, continuing a vicious cycle of endless second chances. Other team members who have been delivering don't feel valued for their hard work and their ability to keep up with deadlines and deliverables. You've been in so many harsh work environments that you've ended up on the other end of the spectrum, creating a different kind of toxicity. In the end, you realize that this employee never intended to perform well but took advantage of your compassion. This situation teaches you that your trust should be earned by actions and not just words.

As you separate who you are from what you do, especially on behalf of others, remember to exercise self-compassion. Generations of Black women before us have identified closely with what they did for others. I constantly hear older Black women in our black girls breathing® community tell me how this is the first time they have even considered caring for themselves. In our community, they've learned to identify traumas that had been normalized for them, rediscover interests that they'd stifled and thought unimportant for so long, and release the belief that they have to come to everyone's rescue. As they adopt new practices for the first time, they applaud the younger women in our community for starting their healing journey earlier. I'm just proud that all these women started, regardless of their age. Let that serve as a reminder to you that it's never too late for you to choose a new story of who you'll be and how you'll show up in the world.

GO-DEEPER EXERCISE: COMMITMENT TO SELF-CARE

It takes intentional work to undo years of programming and redirect your focus from caring for others to caring for yourself. These reflection prompts and the body-scan exercise that follows are a good place to start.

You can journal responses to these prompts all at once or break them up over the course of several sessions. Do whatever feels best for you.

- The greatest resistance I experience when it comes to slowly stripping away my identity as a caretaker is _____ _____.

- I feel like I would most disappoint _____ [name person or people] if I were to change the way I show up for them.

- When I consider the possibility of disappointing that person(s), I think _____.

- I can slowly begin prioritizing myself and my needs in my daily life in these three ways: _____ _____.

- I can commit to trying at least one of those things by _____ [insert date] for _____ [insert time duration].

- As you wrap up this exercise, affirm yourself with the following statements whenever you need:
  - *I give myself permission to choose me.*
  - *I have the tools I need to deal with any shifts in my relationships as I prioritize myself.*
  - *Making time for myself is an act of self-preservation and self-love; it is not selfish.*
  - *I give myself grace for all the times I did not show up on my own behalf in the past.*
  - *Today, I get to make a different decision about who I will be in the world.*

SOMATIC PRACTICE: RESTFUL BODY SCAN

Allowing yourself to rest when your body and mind are usually busy takes practice. Tap in to this body-scan exercise as another rest practice in your arsenal to reframe your identity from being a caretaker to a human being deserving of rest and care.

1. As recommended in chapter 2, be intentional about preparing your space for rest. Draw your blinds or curtains. Light your favorite candle. Turn on some soothing music or use this practice to get comfortable with silence. Get your favorite blanket or comforter. Lie down on your bed, couch, or floor (if this feels accessible to you; if not, feel free to sit). Gently close your eyes or gaze at an object directly in front of you.

2. Begin to draw your attention to the top of your head, where a warm white light will guide you through checking in with each body part to alleviate any tension.

3. From the top of your head, make your way down to your neck, shoulders, and each part of your body until you get to your toes and the bottom of your feet. Allow the white light to help you tune in to how each body part feels. Note any sensations or feelings that arise without judgment.

4. End the practice by giving yourself a big hug as you rock side to side and allow your body to do what it needs to do to feel at ease. Just lie there doing nothing and getting comfortable doing nothing.

Chapter 5

HEALING OUR SISTERHOOD

IF YOU TAKE a look back through African American history, you'll find that we have always gathered. When we are together—at beauty salons, barber shops, corner cookouts, and churches—we experience healing through shared conversations and experiences. At the same time, many of us have experienced trauma caused by someone who looks like us. We owe it to ourselves to explore and heal that pain so we don't pass it on, or worse—avoid deep, intimate relationships with other Black women due to past hurts.

When we've tackled healing as a sisterhood within our black girls breathing® sessions or sunday balm® platform, the depth of trauma has been complex and nuanced. Participants would often become uncomfortable with the idea of addressing trauma that arose from within the community because we were so used to experiencing trauma at the hands of people outside of our community.

But what happens to our views of others and ourselves when we harbor negative thoughts and beliefs about other Black women because of the trauma we've experienced? Perceiving each other in a negative light will foster self-hatred, shame, and a host of other detrimental frameworks that do not move the healing of ourselves and our community forward. In addition, our tradition of gathering that has always been a core part of our identity as a community will slowly die. In order to heal individually and in community, we must tackle those negative thought patterns and perceptions about each other that have been internalized.

We are also still grappling with the pandemic and how it wreaked havoc on our sense of community and changed how we connect with other people. I witnessed a longing for community and the realization that we'd taken for granted opportunities to gather in the past. Suddenly, the person who always used to have a packed schedule, hopping from work to social events to part-time schooling, had the time to be still and reflect on how connecting with others had been not only a form of self-care, but sometimes also a distraction from having to sit with uncomfortable feelings and truths about herself and her sense of identity. At the height of the pandemic, she was forced to become accustomed to stillness and rethink the ways she'd related to others as a means to avoid reckoning with herself.

I've encountered many women like the one I just described who would be skeptical at first about joining a breathwork session for just Black women. She was used to aligning herself to nearly all-white spaces, which clashed with her rising urge to reexplore community with other Black women. After her first session, she would have to sit with her initial hesitance and negative expectations about joining a healing event with women whose experience in the world reflected hers. Why had she had such negative beliefs about her own people? Why did she feel so comfortable in situations where she was one of only a few Black women but not in environments where she was one of many? She was not alone in this experience, but I've often witnessed—in virtual and in-person sessions alike—the walls of skepticism slowly melt away. They unlearn internalized beliefs about other Black women while witnessing firsthand the immense healing of sharing an experience with them that is affirming and uplifting. Slowly, they begin to see that their previous negative experiences with other Black women were influenced by societal conditioning that Black women must compete for limited resources and feel better than one another in order to maintain their sense of security in the world. This phenomenon is often experienced by Black women feeling like they're being "sized up" by another Black woman who doesn't acknowledge their presence with eye contact or warmth but instead evaluates their appearance from head to toe and/or their accomplishments in relation to her own. It's heartbreaking to be on the receiving end of this judgmental energy, especially when it reinforces deeply embedded negative beliefs that Black women are incapable of genuine friendships and sisterhood with each other because of past traumatic experiences.

Internalized racism that makes us think less of ourselves can be a barrier in experiencing sisterhood with other Black women. It's normal to feel a sense of shame for having negative perceptions of people who look like you. I want to affirm your experience as you unlearn—understanding the truth of your beliefs in order to change your thinking, heal from the past, and relate to others in new, beautiful, and healthy ways.

> As you're reading this, you may feel internal objections arise that sound like *I've never experienced this! That's not true! All of my relationships with other Black women have been healthy.* This is a great opportunity to ground yourself with one of our breathwork exercises and recognize that this phenomenon may not apply to *you* and *your experience.* (And even then, this section can encourage you to further explore any blind spots you previously may not have realized you had.) But I've seen it enough while working with thousands of Black women that it was important for me to address and provide tools for us to heal and move forward, sis. It's my goal with this book to bring awareness to certain topics and look directly at realities that might make us uncomfortable in order to bring them into the light for us to address and heal.

HEALING OUR RELATIONSHIPS WITH OTHER BLACK WOMEN

When I dove deeper into sources of hurt stemming from each other in the Black community, I noticed a few things. The traumatic event, like most experiences that cause psychological and emotional wounds, likely happened in childhood or during a formative experience. Maybe you experienced colorism as a darker-skinned Black woman and were discriminated against, othered, and/or made to feel unattractive based on the actions or comments of others when you were growing up ("Oh, you're pretty for a dark-skinned girl"). Or maybe when you got your first job in a mostly white work environment, you expected guidance and support from the only seasoned Black woman there, but she saw you as competition and went out of her way to sabotage your growth and opportunities. Both examples involve experiencing what we expect of an oppressor from someone with brown skin. We expected someone who looked like us to make us feel seen, supported, and celebrated, but we experienced the opposite, which left us feeling rejected with worse emotional pain than if someone outside of our community had done this to us, impacting our sense of self and feeling of belonging. Until we do the healing work to avoid bringing those painful experiences into new environments, we'll continue to project them onto new, promising relationships and communities, sabotaging opportunities to find common ground and an emotional home with other Black women.

Experiencing rejection from another Black woman likely came as a shock to you unless you saw similar dynamics play out in your childhood—for example, in the way your mother or other women in your family spoke of other Black women. It can be so startling and traumatic to experience the opposite of what you expected from another Black woman that you might initially gaslight yourself because you'd rather be wrong about her intentionally hurting you. Even after she has proven to be untrustworthy, you may continue to engage with her, somehow hoping for a different outcome. I've seen this happen most frequently in relationships that we may feel we can't opt out of—like with our families and childhood friends we've trauma bonded with.

Though I cannot speak from personal experience, only from encounters with other women in my work, I've witnessed particularly acute harm when a mixed woman, who self-identifies as Black and has a mother who is white, hears her mother express negative views of Black women during her childhood. This causes her to question her identity and sense of belonging in a way that a mixed, self-identifying Black woman whose mother is Black does not experience.

When it comes to addressing these kinds of issues within our community, we first have to work through the shame that comes with awareness before we can begin the deeper, internal work to heal. Given that so many of us are committed to our internal healing work, there's also an increased desire to be in community with other Black women doing the same. We deserve to heal and thrive not only as individuals but also in our relationships with one another. It is difficult to acknowledge the deep pain that exists in our relationships with each other because this also requires us to admit to the traumas our community has experienced and continues to experience, over hundreds of years. Even as we fight to keep our history from being erased, we also yearn to identify with more than just our pain. Yet we still have to confront our pain head-on.

The more I explored the trauma of rejection within our own

community, the more I realized how common it is among Black women, myself included. Further healing required intensive introspection; with awareness came healing.

CONTEXTUALIZING THE BETRAYAL

If you've experienced harm by another Black woman, it's important to recognize the cognitive dissonance that comes with reflecting on the incident. You may experience disbelief at the lack of support and camaraderie and, in some cases, the betrayal coupled with an understanding of the systemic racism that contributes to this dynamic by instilling self-hatred in us. In a society that perpetuates the belief that there are limited resources and space for people who look like us, it's no wonder that those who find themselves on top subscribe to that myth and work overtime to protect their position from anyone who could potentially take their coveted spot.

While we don't want to justify the harmful actions of another Black woman, it is necessary for our healing to recognize the broader system that contributes to this behavior. Keep in mind that this is for your own sake, not theirs. When you experience betrayal of any kind, it's normal to ask what about you made this person treat you this way. You might ruminate over all your memories with this person, wondering how you missed the signs or how you could've prevented getting hurt. It's imperative that you equip yourself with the emotional and mental tools to not take on the weight of someone else's insecurities or self-hatred.

Even if you've experienced multiple incidents like this and it would be easy to overgeneralize that all Black women are incapable of having close, intimate relationships with each other, try to keep in mind that your relationships will likely shift the more you rid yourself of these negative beliefs and purposefully seek out community with like-minded and -spirited Black women. We exist and it's important that we find each other because the world is hard enough on us.

By slowly moving away from that negative narrative and contextualizing it within the beliefs perpetuated by society, we help the younger version of ourselves who experienced that trauma to heal.

REWRITE THE NARRATIVE

What is your earliest memory of being hurt by another Black woman? Do you remember how that situation made you feel initially? Perhaps you felt shock and confusion, and then those emotions slowly morphed into anger, which turned to sadness as you mourned the relationship you thought you had.

Can you recall what her actions made you believe about yourself and your worth—whether in terms of your intelligence, your appearance, etc.? We must unlearn these negative beliefs in order to reframe how we see ourselves and other people and form healthier relationships. That said, did you have similar traumatic experiences with other Black women? How have you perpetuated this dynamic in your current relationships? For example, if you are used to "friends" who make snide remarks and put-downs disguised as jokes, you might continue to develop relationships with other Black women who reinforce a negative understanding that that type of behavior is a normal part of sisterhood. Consistently experiencing this dynamic then solidifies the false narrative that uplifting and positive relationships with other Black women are impossible, rather than leading you to examine why you feel comfortable and "at home" in relationships with high levels of toxicity. However, when you're able to identify where that first wound from another Black woman came from, you can form new beliefs that help you open yourself up to relationships with Black women that are healthy. You'll know how to identify and steer clear of toxic dynamics and lean in to sisterhoods whose healing disrupts internalized racism. It'll take some conscious and intentional healing work to get from unhealthy to healthy relationships, but it will be oh so worth it in the end.

HEALING IN BEING SEEN

Even though it can feel comforting to embrace isolation after experiencing betrayal, there is an immense amount of healing in allowing ourselves to be seen by others, especially by people who share similar cultural experiences. However, it also requires courage to open ourselves up after being hurt. Though we may do the healing work to get through the bulk of the trauma, the more vulnerably we share with others, the more potential there is to be hurt. But the opposite of making ourselves vulnerable is shutting down and leaning in to avoidance, which robs us of the experience of having valuable connection. Suppressing our innate desire to be a part of a community out of fear of being hurt is such a repressive way to live.

If we live in isolation, it's easy to get caught up in negative mental and emotional spirals and allow our fears to go unchecked. When we engage with our community, we live healthier, happier lives, knowing that we're not alone and receiving support when we need it. Our personal communities can encourage and affirm us when we sometimes ponder,

Am I crazy to feel this way?

Is there something wrong with me?

My life feels fulfilling, but sometimes, honestly, I get lonely.

I'm so emotional. I can't even pinpoint what the problem is. It just feels like everything in my life is in disarray.

What's going on and why is my body responding this way?

When you can see your experience through the eyes of others, it neutralizes harmful thoughts that foster feelings of shame, which tend to spread like wildfire in isolation. The words of support repeated during our black girls breathing® sessions become manifest when we look around the room or the video call and see the shared struggles, grief, joy, and growth experienced by other Black women.

You are not alone.

You have everything you need within.

You are inherently worthy, and there is nothing wrong with you.

And when we as Black women in particular are in community, vulnerably sharing, allowing ourselves to remove the armor that we've had to wear out in the world, we experience an acceptance of our truest selves, with the love of a sisterhood reflected back to us. The more we peel back the layers of protection we've worn out in the world after betrayals, the greater our longing to be seen grows, without titles or pretenses, simply granting ourselves the permission to be uninhibited.

When we consider the realities that we are often the only ones who look like us at our jobs, we don't see ourselves in media representations of beauty, and we experience so many microaggressions in a day, it is an act of resistance to create our own safe space. In fact, I'm reminded that separation was a powerful tool used during slavery. If slave owners could prevent us from gathering, sharing stories and encouraging each other, or dreaming together about what freedom could look and feel like, then they could prevent any uprising through their oppression.

So, our ancestors improvised on the fields, creating songs that helped them get through the workday. They used the allotted time away from the fields on Sundays to imagine a heaven where they could experience relief from their pain and woes. When we do our part to heal from past traumas, our ancestors' dreams are being realized. And though Western culture promotes more individualist ways of thinking and living, we can unlearn self-centered practices and beliefs and return to our roots by prioritizing communal care.

THE 80/20 RULE

The 80/20 rule is a popular concept when it comes to relationship advice. According to this guideline, if your partner has 80 percent of the qualities and values that matter most to you, you should focus on those rather than the 20 percent that might be lacking. We want our relationships to be balanced in terms of giving and receiving one's needs and creating intimacy through vulnerability and transparency with the space to grow and evolve together. Drawing on my personal and professional experiences, I've adapted the 80/20 rule to the context of creating a sense of sisterhood and community while also balancing personal needs.

Before I dive into my version of the 80/20 rule, I want to pause and address how the prevalence of conversation around therapy and mental health has sometimes led to the misapplication of certain concepts. For example, setting boundaries is the subject of many social media posts (#socialmediatherapy), but it can be taken to an extreme so that people veer to an unhealthy level of isolation and develop avoidant behavior patterns rather than the intended goal of boundary setting, which is to encourage secure attachment behaviors and sustain healthy, balanced, ever-evolving relationships. Unhealthy boundary setting creates the expectation that "I don't owe anyone anything" and "I don't need anything from anybody," serving to normalize the sort of toxic independence that undermines the power of genuine community.

Equating strong boundaries with living in total isolation can backfire, as we all need a sense of community and belonging. My adaptation of the 80/20 rule balances a focus on creating a strong sense of self, setting boundaries, and prioritizing personal needs 80 percent of the time with a willingness to be inconvenienced and attend to the needs of your community 20 percent of the time. It is within that 20 percent that the magic of connection happens. This 80/20 rule helps you to simultaneously honor your own needs and make space for genuine community. When you get outside of your comfort zone and invite others to join you on your life's journey, you may be surprised by how rich those connections can be.

What's a boundary that you may have implemented that lacks any flexibility? If you desire to build connection, is this boundary helping you do that? How can you get out of your comfort zone and rigid ways of operating in order to prioritize more connection?

Introverted people and folks dealing with past traumas related to being in community in particular may encounter resistance to forming new friendships and connecting with other Black women. They may think,

I don't have any female friends. You can't trust them.

I've experienced other people being jealous of me and that's why I prefer keeping to myself.

I've been hurt so many times before. I don't want to make myself vulnerable again. It's safer to not bother trying.

When we look at the source of those pains and hurts, it's understandable why this may be your reaction. But I want you to know that there is so much power in being witnessed in community, and it's worth doing the work to move past previous betrayals.

If you encounter resistance, I encourage you to let down your guard a bit and be energetically open to connection. And no, I'm not telling you to pour out your heart to the first potential friend you meet. I'm just saying that you can take small risks while out in public to express openness to community, genuine connection, and the possibility of getting to know another sister intimately. My suggestions may seem inconsequential, but you'd be surprised by how hard this is for many of us who are learning to open ourselves up to new connections.

Practice enjoying your own company. Invest in your hobbies and try to connect with others who share the same interests. I hear a lot of Black women complain that while they are trying to disentangle their sense of identity from their work, it's often the first question that comes up in social settings, so they feel pressured to prove their worth by what they do. This is especially common in certain environments like networking events, so make a conscious effort to be in spaces where the primary purpose is to learn, have fun, and explore. It's also important to try out new things on your own. Many Black women tell me that they have a long list of things they want to explore but they are waiting for the right time or for something else to fall into place first. What if you released all those timelines and expectations and tried those activities regardless of whether you are in a relationship, have lost weight, made more friends, etc.? Allow yourself to explore more of life in your own company. By developing a deeper level of contentment on your own, you create space and opportunity in your life to invite others to join you on the journey you're already enjoying. You tend to attract what you embody internally.

GRADUALLY BUILDING TRUST IN COMMUNITY

A lot of us suffer from toxic hope and empathy. I define toxic empathy as our ability to overlook someone's current behavioral patterns because we have so much compassion for them, given past traumas and experiences that caused those traumas. Rather than recognizing that a person may not be able to meet your needs based on their actions in the present moment, you justify their behaviors and see their potential. They might not even be aware of their own behaviors, much less be able to work through those problems. Even when you do not see them working on their issues right now, you project onto them your hopes for their growth and trust them with more than you should, given their track record, abandoning your own needs in the process. Do you see how this can be a disservice to you and all your hard healing work?

As you intentionally build your community, it's okay to take your time and vet someone or a group before investing fully. In fact, by doing so, you honor yourself and all of the healing you've been doing to reestablish your sense of self-worth after experiencing harm. As you cultivate new connections, listen to your body (i.e., your gut or intuition) when entering new environments and evaluate others' words, actions, and how they show up in different situations and treat others. And as you vet others, it's equally important to open yourself to the possibility of the connections you hope for.

AN EXERCISE FOR UNLEARNING TOXIC EMPATHY

Big, open, and kind hearts are deserving of protection. Navigating past betrayal and traumas you've experienced while in community can make you hesitant to remain as kind and loving as you are in the future. You may be tempted to go to the opposite side of the spectrum, vowing to not be as giving and shutting down that caring aspect of yourself in future interactions. Instead of operating in that extreme, how can you temper certain tendencies you have to project who you are onto others before they've shown themselves to be trustworthy over time? Take some time to evaluate some of the ways you've had toxic empathy in the past. Looking back, where could you have slowed down and stopped projecting all of your good attributes onto another before they actually exhibited those qualities? Come up with two or three ways you'll allow others to reveal themselves gradually over time in the future, as well as appropriate ways to show up in their lives in accordance with what you are witnessing without overgiving. For example, if you tend to overshare intimate details too quickly in new relationships, before the other person has proven to be trustworthy (which is sometimes a subconscious, insecure attachment behavior meant to quickly form a bond), you can create new guidelines for yourself to share appropriate details within certain timeframes (e.g., what is acceptable information to share in the first thirty or sixty days of knowing someone versus six months of knowing them). While curbing the habit of oversharing, you can also think about how an emotionally secure and trustworthy individual will respond to what you share. Observing the other person's responses will show you whether and how much to invest in the relationship, rather than trusting blindly or giving too much in an attempt to create a dynamic that does not exist.

FOSTERING A WELCOMING ENERGY

As a Black woman, you can likely recall many experiences when you've walked into an environment and did not feel welcome. No words had to be uttered in order for you to feel this way because you picked up on the nonverbal cues that communicated that the space was not inviting. As you vet the spaces and people who feel inviting to you, how can you ensure that you're also giving off a welcoming energy so that you're approachable to those who want to get to know you?

If you're extremely introverted or working on overcoming social anxiety (I think we've all had to readjust to in-person connection after experiencing the seclusion of the COVID-19 pandemic), it can be helpful to start with the basics of fostering an inviting energy:

Smile. I winced a bit even writing this, given how often we Black women have heard this command from men who are trying to coerce us into romantic interest. But in the context of trying to meet new friends, a smile is a visual cue that communicates to others, *Hey! I appreciate your presence in this space, and I'd be interested in getting to know you better!*

Practice making eye contact. Nothing feels more like a dagger to the heart than when I'm out in public, usually feeling like "the only" in that environment, and I try to lock eyes with the first Black girl I see, only for her to avoid meeting my eyes and instead size me up with an "up and down" glance. I take the hint that she's not looking for connection (no matter how brief—I was just recognizing your presence, sis!), and I keep it moving. Even if making eye contact is something you have to practice, it communicates directly, *I see you*. Beyond communicating an openness to meeting someone new, eye contact expresses that you are emotionally present, listening, and available to someone. (If it doesn't come naturally, practice in the mirror [revisit the "Mirror Work" section in chapter 2] and in relationships in which you already feel safe so it'll be easier to get in the habit of doing so with strangers.)

Appear physically open. Cultivate a welcoming energy by how you position your body in public. This includes uncrossing your arms and positioning your chest, shoulders, hips, and feet toward anyone you'd like to talk to or are already talking to; maintain a comfortable distance apart, noticing any boundaries that person may be exhibiting that show how closely they feel comfortable engaging with you. Immunocompromised people may keep a good distance between you and them to protect their health, and they may do so by taking a few steps back when you approach them. Try not to take this personally! Make sure you maintain an open stance if you're talking to more than one person (be mindful of not physically closing someone out of the conversation).

CREATE THE COMMUNITY YOU WANT

True community cannot exist if one person is always in the position of receiving. As we balance our overgiving natures, it's important not to go too far to the opposite extreme. Although it feels good to be around givers who make you feel seen and heard, be intentional about cultivating greater awareness so you don't end up taking their kind nature for granted, expecting that person to always show up as the supporter without reciprocating those qualities yourself. You don't want to be the person in a group who takes advantage of the others' kindness and exhibits no interest in developing those same qualities. So how can you be a better community member and friend?

Don't be a passive receiver. No matter how many times your friend says she's low maintenance, create your own personal baseline for how you wish to treat everyone in your sisterhood. Exert the same level of energy for the friend who likes to go on vacation for her birthday every year as you would for the friend who doesn't think her birthday is a big deal but constantly shows up for others' birthdays in a big way. She may not be used to receiving from her friends or anyone in her life. How can you create a more balanced relationship dynamic in your friendship? Observe your friend, notice how she makes others feel valued, and make a conscious effort to mirror these same behaviors back to her. And eventually, depending on where she is on her healing journey, you can even make space for an open conversation where you acknowledge the role she's been playing in your life and communicate that you'd like to do the same for her. Ask what she'd like to see in your friendship to feel equally valued.

Pick up the torch of facilitating gatherings. When you were growing up, you may have seen your parent, aunt, uncle, or guardian demonstrate what it meant to participate in community—for example, by hosting Sunday brunches, Thanksgiving and Christmas dinners, or summer cookouts. We may have participated in these traditions as children without realizing how much effort was involved in hosting, but we always looked forward to partaking in those occasions. I often see a longing for these kinds of gatherings, so as your elders get older, I encourage you to pick up the torch and create these kinds of healing spaces for your family and friends. In addition to family traditions, you can create new traditions among your friends and sisterhood based on your shared interests, like an annual themed party, monthly dinners hosted at a different friend's home each month, or book clubs. You can experience more of the warm, fuzzy feelings that come with being among the people you love by being more intentional about facilitating spaces for everyone to gather instead of waiting for others to host.

Extend grace, understanding, and forgiveness to one another. As someone who is routinely creating safe spaces for Black women to gather and heal, I often encounter the misconception that healing together means there will never be any friction in the group. In order to heal, we often explore triggering topics like our traumas head-on. It's easy to revert to the black-and-white thinking that's so common these days, especially on social media, when we're discussing these topics. This makes it all the more important not only to hear what other people are saying, but to try to understand their lived experience and point of view, in order to live in community together. Avoid jumping to conclusions, think the best of people you're in community with, and do the hard work of maintaining those relationships—offering forgiveness when necessary, asking to be forgiven when necessary, and providing as many chances to your sisterhood as you did your ex (oopsies—JK, sis!).

No matter the experiences that left you feeling hopeless about connecting with other Black women, I hope that the failed attempts and betrayals of the past no longer hold you back from the possibility of experiencing the great joy of being seen in the context of Black sisterhood.

GO-DEEPER EXERCISE: *MORE OF THAT, PLEASE!* VISUALIZATION

This chapter provided several tools to help you evaluate and address the false beliefs you have after experiencing harm from another Black woman, but I want to take this opportunity to help you visualize the soft and caring relationships you desire for the future.

Prepare a peaceful and warm environment for this practice. You can soothe all of your senses by lighting a candle that smells divine, dimming the lights, getting comfy lying down on your bed or the floor or sitting on your couch, and having a sip of your favorite warm beverage beforehand. Gently close your eyes if you feel comfortable doing so. Imagine yourself in the near or distant future. You just got some amazing news that you've been working toward for a long time. Imagine calling a sistah-friend you're in close community with to share the news (whether you currently know this person or are envisioning the friend you're calling into your life). She can't contain her excitement on the phone; she screams, cries, and tells you, "Congratulations," over and over again. She then tells you to get off the phone and get dressed, as she's going to gather the rest of your sisterhood so you all can celebrate that evening. Sinking deeply into that visualization, how does it feel in your body to be seen in this way? What are the feelings that arise? How can you hold on to those feelings as you make space for this reality to arrive? Or better yet, how can you communicate your need to be celebrated to your current community, if you do find your community to be safe? How can you be intentional to seek more positive dynamics like these with other Black women? And how can you make sure you're also cultivating those dynamics in your friendships? The goal of this exercise is to quite literally invite more of these interactions with your energy—sending out a literal signal of *More of that, please!*

SOMATIC PRACTICE FOR RELEASING ANGER AFTER BETRAYAL

Common emotions that arise in the body after experiencing betrayal are anger (toward the other party/parties and self), regret, and disappointment. In addition to breathwork, which is a great tool to not only witness emotions stuck in your body but also work through processing them, there are a few tools that seem elementary and are easily overlooked but work wonders for releasing stagnant and repressed energy from the body.

Yelling: I encourage the use of one's voice in a breathwork session to release emotions like anger that are especially difficult for

Black women to embody due to conditioning. Can you recount the last time you screamed or yelled (not toward others but as a form of release)? If not, your body may be craving it. Whether it's while you're doing a breathwork exercise (after the yell, returning back to the breath can be soothing for your nervous system) or when you need a release in the middle of your day, find a comfortable space, either lying down or sitting. Grab a pillow or a blanket (for consideration of neighbors and as a way to feel comfortable screaming with all of your might) and give yourself a count to three and scream into your pillow/blanket. Feel your stomach completely empty of any emotion into your yell. Repeat as many times as needed until you feel resolved, imagining any of the anger from past betrayals leaving your body with each belt. Make sure to return to a soothing practice of some sort after this activity (e.g., lying down and doing nothing, an oceanic breathwork practice, etc.).

Physical movement: Moving your body is another tool that helps release particularly difficult emotions such as anger and regret. You can opt for creating a playlist that helps you channel some of that anger (many community members have mentioned trap and drill music helping them tap in to their anger better) and try dance, running, or lifting some weights in the gym. As with the yelling exercise, use your chosen physical activity to envision the heavier emotions tied to your past experiences of betrayal leaving the body with each move. Prior to doing the activity, choose a time when your intention is specifically connecting with that anger for the duration of the activity. Commit to feeling it fully, no matter how heavy the emotion feels and intensifies—a normal occurrence—as the time progresses. With physical movements, you can further strengthen the mind-body connection that is also strengthened in consistent breathwork practice.

No matter your past experiences, I'm wishing you beautiful sisterhoods and community ahead, sis!

Chapter 6

DREAMING BRAVELY

THE OPTION TO think beyond our day-to-day struggles feels like a luxury for many Black women. Our position in the world is such that we have to invest so much energy into taking care of our bodies and health and showing up for our careers and those around us that having energy left over is a miracle. So many of us are simply trying to survive. But as this book helps you unlearn this conditioning to not prioritize yourself or your dreams, my hope is that you'll dare to dream. I say "dare to dream" because our struggle is not just on an individual level to feel more free, but also with a world that combats our freedom. We see this in how many Black women who are thriving and excelling as they live out their dreams are punished for their audacity to be excellent and authentic. These women range from Beyoncé and Serena Williams to Claudine Gay, a Black woman thriving in academia who was questioned about her experience and her career path (with the assumption that she had it easier than the average person because she must have become Harvard University president through affirmative action or DEI efforts). We are constantly being held to higher standards than our non-Black peers.

So, as I encourage you to dream bravely, know that I am aware that it will come with some fight. It will come with a kind of effort that none of your non-Black colleagues will be able to relate to as you climb higher and higher. Knowing and accepting this reality makes it all the more important for you to armor yourself with the tools presented in this book. You cannot dream as a Black woman without a strong sense of self, a guiding light, and a personal community to pour back into you when the world switches from applauding your hard work for filling in the gaps and raising the bar in your industry to suddenly perceiving you as a threat. "How did she even get here?" "She must have been a diversity hire." "You know they're giving a bunch of grants to Black women now."

Black girl, your dreams are a threat. I know that's not the warm and fuzzy feeling you were expecting when you picked up this book, but it is our reality. And instead of setting false pretenses for a Black girl who dreams fiercely and unapologetically, I want to make sure you are well equipped. Your ability to manifest dreams that our ancestors sacrificed for by making it to another day is one thing, but building up the strength to protect that dream once you've accomplished it is another. It's so important that we are prepared for all that will be required for a Black woman to actualize her dreams. But despite the fear that may arise when you recognize that you may be met with hostility for daring to dream, both within and outside of our community, I'm still advocating for you to go for it anyway. Because I'll be damned if our ancestors were brave enough to survive the cotton fields in hopes of a better, more just future, only for us to give up now. Sis, it won't be easy, but I truly believe it will be worth it—not just for us but for all the little Black girls who will come after us.

Before you dive into some explorative healing work for your inner child/teenager/young adult/younger version of you, let's take a deep inhale and exhale. Reading up to this point in the chapter may have triggered some sad and heavy feelings about the reality of being a Black woman and the obstacles to living outside the small boxes the world has put you in. I know. I hear you; I see you. Close your eyes, feel yourself sink deeper into whatever surface is supporting you, and inhale into your nose slowly, filling every area of your lungs, then exhale out of your mouth. Repeat three times and come back to the rest of the chapter when you feel ready.

UNEARTHING OR REMEMBERING YOUR DREAMS

We all have dreams. And if reading that statement triggers self-doubt, I want you to know that even if your dream has been buried by all of life's injustices and disappointments, it's still there. It just might take you some time to rediscover and breathe new life into it, especially as you see beyond your traumas and past experiences and as you imagine all that a healed you can be. You do have a dream and you are worthy of seeing that dream come to pass.

Recall the first dream or goal you remember having. What

age were you, and is there anything else you remember happening in your life at the time? Did you ever pursue that dream later on in life? Why or why not? If that dream is still on pause because you are waiting for the perfect conditions to start or you became overwhelmed with what it would take to realize it, let's dive deeper into how we can break those dreams down into smaller, actionable steps.

DAILY ACTIONS TO TURN DREAMS INTO A REALITY

Start small. Any big goal requires mustering up self-belief as you achieve tiny goals that help you realize that not only is your larger goal attainable, but that you, the person carrying out the dream, have all you need to see it through. A big dream doesn't require you to foresee at the beginning how every tiny step and detail in the process will play out to get you to your end goal. (That's an impractical way to see the world and will inhibit you from ever starting something new.) A big dream requires you to be open and willing to start the process and explore. Once you honor the call, your dream(s) will present a journey in which you discover the right information, meet the right people, and even make the needed mistakes. Yes, I said "mistakes" because all those elements working together will cumulatively get you closer to reaching your end goal.

When it comes to accomplishing a goal, it's important to deeply identify with or become the type of person you'll need to be in order to reach that goal. This is less about trying to become someone you're not and more about developing the types of behaviors and skills needed to see that dream through. If your dream is to become a doctor, you'll need to manage an intense study schedule and learn how to study properly. If your dream is to own a business providing a service to clients, whether it's helping people find their dream home as a real estate agent or having the most trusted brokerage firm, you'll need to develop your selling and people skills. The list goes on. Once you've identified the kinds of qualities you need to reach a particular goal, you'll want to find ways to practice those qualities day by day until they become habitual and eventually second nature to you.

A common mental block that arises when someone begins to get serious about the future they want to create for themselves is feeling like they don't have enough time to establish new routines. Notice how I used the word *feeling* instead of stating as a fact that they don't have enough time to practice a consistent habit day by day. Often, it is a feeling that they have perceived as true for so long that it now has the same effect as a fact. But if you always feel you don't have time, the question is, when will you?

To unlearn this belief of not having enough time, start by making small changes that may not be directly connected to your goal. I implement this technique in direct response to the doubts I experience around working toward my goals. For instance, perhaps you'd like to get in the habit of keeping your living space tidier or cooking at home more often. Keeping a clean space may not look like it's directly related to building that business you want, but do you notice how much better you feel and work when you keep a tidy space? A clean work area now gives you more mental space to focus on your work so you're more productive with your time. Or maybe you want to increase your physical activity. At first glance, the goal doesn't seem to be tied to getting your brokerage license, but a consistent workout routine will increase your energy and provide you with the stamina needed to reach your goal. You see where I'm going here? If you allow the narrative of not having enough time to direct your choices in life, it will be impossible to find the wherewithal to accomplish things that exist outside your usual routine.

For whatever activity you choose to practice this technique with, measure how long the activity actually took and note how you felt once you finished the task and what you learned about yourself or the task in the process. This reflection will help you to be more present in any undertaking and see that no matter how inconsequential an activity may seem, you can always learn something new. In fact, many of your "aha" moments come when you've made space to have a clear and focused mind. You'll discover that you can easily take time away from mindless tasks to focus on goals that you didn't think you had time for. For example, you may have figured out that it takes you thirty minutes to walk a mile. When you examined your daily routine, you realized that you normally spend thirty-five minutes scrolling TikTok during your lunch break. Now that you have this information, you might decide to eat your lunch and then go on a one-mile stroll instead of scrolling social media so you can reach your goal of exercising more. Although I've used this example, I also want to be mindful of the fact that sometimes we need a healthy distraction to get lost in another world when we deal with so much in a day. "Checking out" is a strategy many of us use to decompress and dissociate from the heavier, more painful things we deal with on a day-to-day basis, and I thoroughly advocate for healthy distractions like comedic content on TikTok, as alluded to in the mental-rest examples listed in chapter 2. As we sprinkle some of those moments throughout our day, we can also be more mindful of how much time we dedicate to those activities compared to the habits needed to accomplish our goals.

Activity/Goal	Amount of Time Needed to Accomplish Goal	Mindless Task That You Can Take Time Away From	Feeling After Completing the Goal	Something I Learned About the Task or Myself After Completing the Goal

Use this process to reframe how you set your goals and be sure to return to this exercise to keep track of what you learn about yourself or the accomplishment. You'll begin to rewire your thought processes and beliefs about what you can accomplish. Once you move past that initial resistance where doubt prevented you from working toward a certain goal (starting with small steps), you'll discover your own capacity to shift your behavior and build your internal muscles to move from smaller goals to larger dreams.

Our dreams exist outside of our comfort zone and the way

we're used to doing things. I'm reminded of the saying "How you do one thing is how you do all things." Becoming your biggest advocate to see your own dreams through will require a sense of mastery of the nonrenewable resource of your time. By better respecting your own time, you'll also become more mindful of how you give your time to others and what you say yes to. You'll become a better steward of your time and simultaneously build better boundaries along the way.

In addition to encouraging you to better manage your time, I want to address another mental block that stops many of us Black women before we even get a chance to start: the idea of perfection. We have a deeply embedded belief that we have to be perfect and our steps have to be perfect or else we are not worthy or well equipped to actualize a dream in the first place. This belief has been reinforced by our society for centuries, and although the belief did not originate within us, we have the opportunity to stop measuring our efforts so harshly and placing unrealistic expectations on ourselves.

RELEASE THE IDEA OF PERFECTION

If I got a dollar for every time I heard the saying "Be twice as good for half as much," I might not need to work another day in my life. That familiar phrase that I grew up hearing planted deep-seated beliefs around the need to constantly prune myself to perfection. Look decent. Talk well. Be the best. Be at the top. Work harder than everyone else if you want to be considered for that opportunity. These were the rules a little Black girl absorbed from parents who were raised during the civil rights era; witnessed integration in Birmingham, Alabama, and Muskegon, Michigan; and learned from watching their own parents and witnessing in real time the effects of racism.

I have a memory from high school that stands out clearly to me. At the time, I was going to a mixed-demographic school—half-white and half-Black—after having attended a nearly all-white high school and middle school. I remember my dad coming to school to check me out for a doctor's appointment. He was not pleased with a middle-of-the-day commitment that would require me to miss school. "This must be the class you have a ninety in," he muttered. That ninety was my lowest grade at the time. You see, I was always a star student. Top of the class. Honor roll with the extracurricular activities to match. Technically, a ninety was still an A, but it wasn't good enough for my dad. It wasn't until I was older that I realized that his comments were not so much a critique of my performance as they were his attempts to prepare me for a world where I would have to be perfect to advance as a Black woman. My teenage self could only perceive and internalize the endless need to be perfect. Through that experience and many others, I learned early on that "not quite" and "almost" were not choices for me as a Black woman. My intelligence and capacity would always be questioned when I showed up in a room, so my credentials and perceived value had to precede me. My path to success would be critiqued by anyone who felt threatened by my presence, my ability to use my voice to take up space, the way my inner light shined, and my directness in expressing my needs and looking beyond what others considered to be more than enough for me, a young Black woman. After all, to them, my disposition should be one of only immense gratitude for any perceived opportunity afforded me, as surely it was a handout and not anything I worked hard for, no matter the reality of the situation. So many of us Black women can relate to this.

Just as we can inherit intergenerational traumas, people can also inherit attitudes and mindsets from their predecessors. If their forefathers handed out scraps while carrying a sense of self-entitlement, these beliefs were passed down to later generations unless they were actively unlearned. So how do we detach ourselves from this cruel game of having to prove our value and overexerting ourselves to our detriment? We stop living up to unrealistic ideals that were founded on unjust systems. Although the injustices may still remain, we have a choice in how we decide to show up in response each and every day.

We have had to take on the weight of the outside world's scrutiny as our own cross to bear, disproving negative perceptions time and time again. And one of the main ways we've done so is by creating for ourselves a standard of perfection. "If I know all aspects of this project and outshine my colleagues, then they will *finally* see my value and my worth." "If they see I can afford all these designer items, then they'll stop discriminating against me when I only want to browse." The scenarios are endless but ultimately boil down to using a standard of perfection as a defense mechanism against others' preconceived notions of who we are. But perfection is a lie, one that's been so ingrained that we even judge younger, more rebellious Black women who have chosen to defy this standard and have done the work to choose another reality. Take a look around and think of all the examples of Black women you know who have chosen differently. How were they received when they decided to operate outside of that framework? Were they not considered outcasts or bad representatives of what a Black woman should be?

We've been so indoctrinated by the concept of perfectionism that we then turn around and project those unrealistic ideals onto younger Black women who, by some miraculous feat, may not have been indoctrinated by this same ideology. But how do we tap in to that young Black girl inside of us, before she adopted this toxic way to present herself and relate to the world? How do we shed this protective layer and the weight of striving to outperform others' bigotries?

The first step is acknowledging that we are, in fact, not perfect. We are human beings having an imperfect human experience. Although the world has not taken into account our humanity, placing the Strong Black Woman trope on us, we get to reclaim our humanity by shifting the narrative and doing the work outlined in previous chapters to redefine who we are in the world and create our own sense of self. Recall the first memory you have of needing to show up perfectly in the world. What were the beliefs you had about yourself at the time? Who communicated to you that you had to show up in this way? How do those words affect you now? Which of those beliefs are no longer serving you or encouraging you to show up as a full human being rather than be hyperfocused on perfection?

PRACTICE MAKING PEACE WITH UNCERTAINTY

The reality of life is that no matter how much we operate as though we have control, we don't. I'm sure you can find many examples in your own life journey when you were knocked off your center. Experiencing the sudden death of someone close to you, being fired from your job or feeling forced to leave because the environment was so toxic that it was beginning to destroy your mental health (many Black women's experience), or receiving a diagnosis that required you to reconfigure your life—whatever the specifics of your situation, you could never have expected or planned for these things. But it's possible to have a healthier relationship with the full spectrum of life experience and release the need to control by making peace with uncertainty instead of fighting against it. The more you're able to ride the waves of unpredictability in your life, the more life you'll be able to live. When you're forced to take it one step at a time while traveling through a dark tunnel, you won't succumb to despair. You'll have the tools and the hope needed to see you through.

Training your brain to be more comfortable with the unknown can begin with simple actions like taking a different route home from work or spending a weekend without a set schedule and driving to a neighborhood you've always wanted to explore, taking a walk, grabbing some coffee at the local coffee shop, and asking the barista about their favorite things to do in the neighborhood. The idea is to get comfortable with not knowing something, navigating a new situation, and making it to the other side so you begin to trust your ability to do so again in the future. Accept the fact that life involves upsets, disruptions, and valley moments. We can get ahead of the curve as much as possible by anticipating those moments and arming ourselves with the tools to navigate through those rough patches.

CREATE AN EVIDENCE LIST

In addition to my faith, my evidence list is a go-to when I'm navigating rough terrain in life. The list is the "proof in the pudding," recounting all the times I made it through despite many fears, doubts, and negative thoughts swirling in my mind. When I continue to encounter moments like these, I meditate on those past experiences, recounting as many details as possible. I use my past evidence to directly counter negative thoughts and affirm my ability to keep journeying, one day at a time. Depending on the season you currently find yourself in, your journey might look like taking care of your daily basic needs (eating several meals a day, drinking enough water, getting sleep, taking a shower) or feeling the pressures mounting as you experience a major transition (like working on your business full-time or getting a promotion and moving to a new city where you don't know anyone). Life will always include some degree of uncertainty. The question remains: How will you navigate it?

> Take some time to reflect on past situations where fears of the unknown were prevalent and jot down what the outcome was and what you learned about your capabilities as a result. These reflections will act as pieces of evidence that

you can make it through uncertain times. This proof of your resilience and innate abilities will remind you that you don't need to know what the future holds all of the time to be able to navigate whatever life brings.

The Situation	Fears That Surfaced During the Time	The Outcome	What You Learned About Your Abilities

MEASURE AND CELEBRATE YOUR PROGRESS

Another effective tool to combat perfectionism as you take steps toward realizing your dreams is to make a habit of consistently recognizing each small win and celebrating your progress along the way. In the context of healing work, it is especially important to see your progress as success; otherwise, whenever you feel triggered, you might be tempted to consider all your healing efforts as unsuccessful because you have a standard of perfection.

Once you develop a consistent habit of noticing your progress, you will be more inclined to think this way about other developing parts of your journey. You'll recognize that the presence of a trigger doesn't indicate a lack of growth but an opportunity to respond differently than you would have in the past. And I would be remiss if I didn't address the fact that you may need to do some unlearning in order to see yourself as worthy of celebration after long having been told otherwise. If you've focused only on external validation for accomplishments in the past, it can take time to even notice, much less celebrate, the quieter victories that only you see. But by tuning in to your own journey, you develop a stronger sense of self and set your own standards of success that aren't dependent on others' perceptions.

THE GOODIE JAR EXERCISE

It's important to collect evidence of your progress and wins and reminders that you're doing just fine to change your frame of reference from an unrealistic standard of perfection and comparison to a daily celebration of your forward movement (even when it doesn't *feel* like it). You can do this exercise digitally (by creating a folder on your phone or computer) or physically (with a mason jar or scrapbook). Begin documenting (by taking a screen shot of the email, picture, text, etc., if you go the digital route or writing on a piece of paper or printing out a physical copy) every time you experience a small or big win. Examples of wins include receiving a compliment for your creativity on a recent project, noticing your improved response to an adverse situation that you would've responded to differently in the past, and successfully keeping promises to yourself (juicing weekly, moving your body several times a week, eating balanced meals) even and especially if you didn't feel like doing them. These goodie jars will be full of helpful reminders at any point when you need a concrete example of your growth, especially when you find yourself in an anxious mental spiral and don't *feel* as if there's been progress. You'll need this tool along your journey as you navigate not only the internal battles but external ones that we, Black women, will unfortunately and undoubtedly face.

PREPARE FOR DISAPPOINTMENTS

Lean in close, sis. If you're doing something that you haven't seen done before, whether it's in your family or workplace, expect mistakes because you learn as you go. Expect some disappointments as you reach for new heights while also having to navigate how the outside world perceives you, a Black woman, reaching for such heights. The question is not *if* there will be disappointments but *when*. And how will you respond so they don't wipe you out and you have the courage to get back up again?

The better you can prepare your mind and spirit to encounter these situations, the better you'll be able to navigate external attacks to your dreams and come out on the other side. Preparation does not mean trying to circumvent normal, human reactions to perceived setbacks and disappointments. We are not robots without feelings. But as the popular saying goes, "We can stay ready so we don't have to get ready." You may be surprised to hear me tell you to prepare for disappointment in an inspirational self-help book, but as a Black woman who is dreaming far bigger than the world has said I'm entitled to, I have to speak authentically and in good faith because I truly care about the betterment of Black women. Disappointment will come, and my prayer is that you will have the tools, the strong sense of self, and the community you need when it does. Know that even as I encourage you to dream big, you are still more than your accomplishments. Your worth and value as a Black woman exist outside of the things you're able to do.

YOUR BAD-DAY TOOL KIT

Identify what makes you feel grounded and reminds you of who you are and your purpose in preparation for bad days. Maybe there is a set of affirmations or a Bible verse or a physical place that makes you feel secure in seasons of uncertainty and instability. These things will vary from person to person, so it's important to know yourself and your needs. You don't need to spend a lot of time trying to figure out what's worked for other people; the cheat code is to focus on what works for you. If you need help figuring out what should be in your bad-day tool kit, start by asking some self-reflection questions:

- What activities and places have helped me feel more secure in moments when I was disappointed or sad? For example, visiting my hometown helps ground me so I can see the big picture in the context of where I came from and just how far I've come. Knitting helps me feel a sense of calm and security when the world around me is spiraling out of control.

- Who in my personal community makes me feel seen and is a safe place for me to share my experiences? For example, my mom always provides a listening ear and doesn't make me feel judged. I can also share when I'm having a hard time in black girls breathing's sunday balm® community without feeling judged or less than.

Tap in to whatever physical or virtual spaces or physical, mental, or emotional tools you need to find refuge when things aren't going according to plan and it feels like too much to bear. And in seasons when you don't need your bad-day tool kit as often, continue to invest in it, especially your personal community. Don't treat your friends and family like an emergency helpline, only engaging when you feel down, as that is a surefire way to weaken those relationships. Go out in the world, Black girl, not only with your big dreams and ambitions, but with a plan to support those dreams when you encounter naysayers and setbacks.

Whatever it is that you have a deep desire to accomplish, I hope the tools in this chapter help you create a foundation to dream and live boldly in the world despite any obstacles that may come your way. I'd like to add that it's important for you to do the healing work necessary to differentiate between a true internal calling and a desire to do something simply because someone else is doing it or because you believe realizing the dream will fill a need for belonging. It won't, sis. You will have to figure out how to fulfill that need for yourself because no dream will give you a sense of identity, worth, and value. Thankfully, that sense of self-worth is not dependent on external circumstances.

GO-DEEPER EXERCISES

Keep yourself accountable for completing the exercises in this chapter. Start by spending thirty minutes or more each week going through one of the exercises. If you have the thought *I don't have time*, or if any resistance in your body comes up, start with the exercise in the "Daily Actions to Turn Dreams into a Reality" section on page 121 to practice reallocating the time you spend on mindless activities to other tasks that better align with your goals.

As you work through some of these activities, big feelings are bound to arise. It's normal, sis. When you think about where you'd like to be, it's easy to become critical of your past, thinking about how you could've incorporated this work sooner and maybe gotten farther along on the path than you are. It's normal to feel this way, but I also want you to understand that we can use past mistakes and mishaps as lessons for the future—we wouldn't have that knowledge and wisdom without those past experiences. So don't punish your past self with today's insights. Give yourself the gift of compassion as you permit all those hard feelings to arise and make space to feel them fully so you can move past them with the breath.

BREATHWORK FOR SELF-COMPASSION: NASAL BREATHING

1. Start by lying on your side in a fetal position (if this is comfortable and accessible to your body; use any soft tools

for support: e.g., pillow, blanket, etc.). As any perfection-istic "should've," "could've," or "would've" thoughts arise, gently embrace yourself, allowing your body to sink into whatever surface is supporting you, and notice your natural breathing pattern.

2. Begin to deepen your natural breathing and inhale and exhale through your nose. Inhaling through your nose with elongated, slow, and deep breaths, feel your chest rise and your rib cage expand. Exhaling out of your nose, feel your stomach hug your rib cage as you deplete your lungs.

3. Allow any feelings of regret and guilt from your past to come to the surface, giving them space to be felt while compassionately releasing them with each exhale. With each inhale, you make space to affirm with pride that you have all the right knowledge at the right time, and you are exactly where you need to be. Happy breathing, sis.

Chapter 7

FINDING FREEDOM DESPITE OPPRESSION

FOR OUR COMMUNITY, thriving has almost always been an internal state. Maintaining a strong sense of self was a saving grace for our ancestors who experienced cruel treatment and oppression. It is essential for Black folks today to continue to cultivate a strong internal sense of freedom, which has helped me to navigate the world as a Black woman and given me the strength and resilience to continue pressing forward with black girls breathing.®

While the field of mental health tends to focus on an individual's perspective and response to their external world, it would be overly simplistic to tell Black people that achieving personal growth and shifting their perspective are enough to alleviate all their traumas and suffering without any consideration of the systems that continue to prevent Black people from being completely free. I would even argue that the fact that Black experience is not truly seen and accounted for in the research and methodologies used by many therapists today contributes to the barriers and distrust that prevent Black people from seeking therapy. To think that a commitment to therapy would alleviate all our problems without addressing the social determinants of our health would be ignorant and naive. Therapy does not fix problems like a lack of financial resources and the struggle to escape generational poverty, or public zoning that prevents Black schools from receiving the same level of resources as other schools in nearby districts. Poor mental health is a natural outcome of living in a constant state of fight or flight because of neighborhood violence or housing insecurity and financial lack. The shackles of slavery and the rules of Jim Crow shape-shifted into a system that sets up more subtle barriers against people who are trying to pull themselves up by their bootstraps, whose only hope in the square radius of their block is their local church or their grandma's house, where Grandma refuses to succumb to the misery and hopelessness around her, evidenced by dilapidated homes that once belonged to a thriving, close-knit Black neighborhood that now frequently loses people a quarter of her age to disease or gun violence.

Through my work, I've been exposed to massive amounts of trauma and pain in our community. Just as I inherited trauma from my predecessors, I also inherited resilience and hope that affirmed to me that despite occasional moments of hopelessness, I am not toiling in vain. My work to provide a safe space for my community to heal may not solve all their problems, but at least it allows them to drop their guards and feel seen and heard in a space that was made just for them. Many of us experience the plight of trying to dream beyond our current harsh realities to a brighter future. For my grandmother's and earlier generations, the pain was so great that heaven was their only hope. Yet we continue to dream of creating a world where our children's children will experience not only a sense of internal freedom, but also freedom manifested in the world around them. One day, it will feel safe to occupy a Black body without hesitancy, fear, or internalized shame. But until that day arrives, we are tasked with protecting our inner peace, joy, and hope in the midst of turmoil. In the words of many older Black church women I've come across, "This joy I have—the world didn't give it, so the world can't take it away."

As you do inner healing work, being able to tap in to internal spaces that are not riddled by trauma is a reality that many of our ancestors could only dream of. It's important for us to take stock of the progress made between generations, as well as within ourselves, to encourage us to keep inching forward, step by step, just like our ancestors did as they survived tragedies to bring us closer to a just world. Until we reach that goal, proactively guard your inner peace that you've worked so hard to cultivate amid ever-recurring traumas in a society that is still uncomfortable with the idea of us being truly free.

NAVIGATING HOPELESSNESS

When you find yourself in a season of personal or collective struggle, when the world is more attuned to the plight of our people (e.g., the rise of the Black Lives Matter movement in the wake of the murders of Sandra Bland, George Floyd, and Breonna Taylor), it's so easy to slip into a state of deep hopelessness. Why bother trying? Why bother showing up and trying to push our communities forward if this is the way it has been for such a long time?

Considering how long we've been enslaved versus free, we may feel hesitant to pursue any ambitions for creating a path forward. How can we dare see a flicker of hope in the midst of such dire circumstances? I'm not asking you to shake that feeling of hopelessness or rush past it in your hurry to feel a sense of hope again; I would never ask you to sidestep any of your emotions. But I am asking you to allow yourself to witness all the thoughts and feelings that arise with that sense of hopelessness, to make space for it and process it. Any glimpse into how Black people around the world are treated and how our dreams and lives have been stolen and cut short could cause a negative spiral. But even as we recognize that dark reality, we also see how our ancestors created their own joy (and were generous enough to let the world partake in it) in the form of their food, their imprint on music (blues, gospel, rock, pop, etc.), and their scientific and technological innovations.

When I find myself in a negative spiral where I'm questioning the impact of my work considering the scale of our problems, I remind myself of my family history. My grandmother only knew grimness, pain, and trauma when she made the decision to leave Money, Mississippi, to seek a better life in the Midwest. I think about how much fortitude she had to move, believing that a better life did exist even though she hadn't seen any evidence of it yet. She had so little on which to base her hope; yet she still found hope. This vision, though costly, is a superpower that has sustained our people and continues to sustain us as we inch toward a better existence. My grandmother had a sense of purpose that motivated her to take action and believe in a future that was almost inconceivable, given her present reality.

RETURNING TO YOUR WHYS

When you encounter yet another news story of police brutality, violence, or injustice toward Black women, or are personally fatigued by another microaggression in the workplace, arming yourself with your deeper whys will give you the strength to zoom out, refocus, and find your center. Spending time doing the work described in the previous chapters will help you identify your whys and rely on them in times of need.

There is a reason why you are doing the difficult healing work of addressing your traumas, both individual and generational, and navigating the grief that comes with them. No matter how fatigued you are, something within you compelled you to pick up this book and do this work. So while your mind and body may feel heavy and hopeless at times, you still have hope buried deep within. Your job now is to find it and hold on to it. Ask yourself these questions:

- *What are my intentions in furthering my healing?*
- *What motivated me to refuse to succumb to "the way things have always been" in my life?*
- *How would I rewrite my personal history if I could?*
- *When it comes to my lineage and the culture to which I belong, how would I rewrite our collective history if I could?*

Your answers to these questions will help guide you to your hope, no matter how deep it is buried within you. The way you would rewrite the history of your culture, your neighborhood, and your family unveils your why. That why is evident in your existence and your efforts to heal and do the work to move the needle forward in your lifetime, no matter how small you perceive that progress to be. Your ancestors planted that seed of your purpose a long time ago, before they could even glimpse our future freedom. And it's our job to keep that hope alive. We remind ourselves of the progress made since our elders' lifetimes and sense the pride that they would feel if they could see us, knowing their fight and resilience were not in vain. To be clear, this does not mean that we overlook the very real and prevalent injustices that continue to impact every aspect of our lives as Black people. Acknowledging our progress does not mean burying our heads in the sand and hoping for the best, but we remember our ancestors' legacy when hopelessness threatens to consume us. Even as you identify your why and the source of your hope, it's okay if it still feels hard to access or fully embody some days. All that matters is that you keep trying in a world that continues to be unfair and harsh toward us.

LEANING ON THE WISDOM OF YOUR ELDERS AND ANCESTORS

Sometimes the individualist mindset of Western societies makes it easy to center our own experiences and feel as though we are the first ones to come up against the challenges of our generation. While our specific obstacles may look different in a world that is more interconnected than ever before, the reality is that our challenges are fundamentally the same as those of our predecessors. Our elders have had similar and perhaps greater fights than what we are navigating today. I'm reminded of how my motivation for creating black girls breathing® was to help us feel seen and not alone by healing in community. Similarly, we recognize that we're not alone in our struggles when we look to those who've come before us and lean on their wisdom, knowledge, and spiritual sustenance.

In a world that seeks to erase our history and ban any books deemed controversial, it is more important than ever before to know your personal and collective history. There have been days when I've been so grateful to live in close proximity to my mom and grandma while doing this work. I get an immense, unspeakable strength just by being in their presence. Their very existences exemplify how to make it through the worst of history and still be able to laugh, find daily reasons to thank God, and be in their right minds. Their poise characterizes many Black women who faced impossibilities and, on the other side of the struggle, "didn't look like what they'd been through." Whether I directly ask about their experiences in the world and glean from their advice and wisdom, or I simply observe how they respond to certain situations, I'm reminded that I am not the first or, as exemplified by our black girls breathing® community, the last to experience these struggles.

As you hear your elders' stories of triumph, ask questions and record this living history, because a battle is being waged against our triumphs and strengths. Recognize that their stories aren't so far removed from ours. Honor their wisdom by being a witness to their story—maybe you are the first person to ask them about it. Take note of their sacrifices. How did they progress? In what ways did they galvanize and collectively effect change? How did they support themselves and each other? What were their versions of "self-care"? What dreams did they not get to realize but hope the generation after them would accomplish? Take note of these responses. Celebrate their tenacity. Jot down the wildest dreams they had that you are currently living. These narratives will serve as proof that our dreams are worth fighting for and that the progress thus far is worth celebrating.

Through our elders' strength and wisdom, we can develop a sense of pride instead of shame that this world would like to put on us when it comes to our history. Growing up, I noticed how there was such a sense of shame when people discussed slavery; now couple that shame with newfound attempts to rewrite history and distance ourselves from those atrocities. In light of these circumstances, we resist any stereotypes associated with our foods and are proud of our wealth of knowledge gained from toiling over the land. We resist any shame and honor the wisdom of our ancestors and pay them reverence. If not for their labor and skill, life as we know it would not exist. In order to embody hope fully, we would do well to rely on our elders' wisdom. We need to understand how they got by and how they got through, as my grandmother would say, "by and by."

IDENTIFYING THE ELDERS IN YOUR LIFE

I'm well aware that not everyone has a healthy enough dynamic with their immediate family to feel comfortable doing some of the exercises in this chapter. However, you can get creative to connect with the elders in your community, whether it's through a local community center where there's programming for the elders in your neighborhood, or you belong to a denomination or church where you can find elders who have much wisdom to impart; many churches were pivotal in the civil rights movement. That older Black woman or man at your job? Introduce yourself, form a relationship, and get to know their life's journey. You most likely will find unparalleled wisdom and stories waiting to be told.

THE VALUE OF COMMUNITY

Individuality is a Western concept that does not serve us when dealing with injustice. As evident in various African cultures today, community is a central source of joy and hope. Community gives us the wherewithal to face challenges out in the world. A lot of time spent in isolation is unhealthy for anyone, but I believe it can be especially damaging for people whose ancestors thrived by living in mutual dependence on each other. Members of the Black Gen X or baby boomer community may recount stories from "back in their day" about how their Black neighborhoods and communities used to interact with each other. The neighbors' kids were like their parents' kids in the way their parents took responsibility for them. People shared their resources. There was a sense of connectivity that outweighed any perceived differences. My grandfather Howell would always share with me that he saw the breakdown of that sense of connectedness when integration began, despite the benefit of new, hard-earned liberties. The beginning of equality and a newfound sense of freedom might have contributed to less of an appreciation for the community that had always sustained us.

CENTERING JOY IN THE MOVEMENT

In times of tragedy in our communities, social media has often been a forum to hold both immense sadness and joy. It isn't uncommon for the world to witness trauma in real time on social media and grieve en masse and then within twenty-four hours of said tragedy, find a meme trending on #BlackTwitter that adds levity to the situation. Responses to the meme are inevitably divided between those who believe that it is evidence of an inability to take traumatic events seriously and those who consider it affirmation that we are a multifaceted people who are able to hold both tragedy and joy at the same time. I believe that our ability to find laughter and joy in the midst of immense tragedy has always been one of our community's greatest strengths. Some of our most prominent inspirations and innovations, from award-winning music to acclaimed literature, have been birthed from pain. We've alchemized trauma into brilliant art, harnessing our rich and joyous legacy in response to whatever may come against us in the world.

If I've learned anything from doing work that exposes me to an immense amount of trauma, it's the importance of prioritizing joy. Our Black existence is so much more than the hardships we've experienced. There are arguments among our community about whether our art forms (film, TV, books) focus too heavily on trauma. I deeply understand the sentiment of not wanting to center our pain, but I also see why these depictions are necessary because the abhorrent realities of our history, some of which happened fairly recently to our parents and grandparents, are at risk of being erased. I also believe that we are all collectively yearning for more joy. We still aren't free and experience daily traumas and microaggressions, which make it all the more important for us to be reminded that life is worth living. The beautiful thing about the range of Black experiences is that Black joy can look different for us all.

Growing up in Atlanta, I experienced Black joy when my mom worked at the 1996 Olympics so I could see Dominique Dawes in real life, when I attended SpelHouse football games and yard shows with my sister during homecoming weekend, and when I participated in annual church lock-ins. In adulthood, I celebrate Black joy by listening to our music, catching up with my sistah-friends in any way I can with our busy schedules (even if it's just during a grocery-store run or nature-trail walk), and scrolling TikToks filled with Black content creators who make me laugh about seemingly universal Black experiences. Centering joy is an essential part of our healing and advancement.

IDENTIFYING YOUR JOYS

While we each find joy in ways that are unique to us, I also encourage you to look for joy that is connected to other Black people and our community as a whole. Given the collective pain we've experienced, it's all the more important to find collective joy. In doing so, we cement our identities in a more well-rounded way that is not based solely on our pain. Take thirty minutes to write down or audio record joys you've experienced within the Black community to remind yourself of modern Black jubilee the next time you are exposed to another tragedy.

ADVOCATING FOR YOURSELF

As you engage in healing work, strengthen your sense of self, and find joy in community, you will be better equipped to advocate for yourself in a society that has historically taken away your agency. I've often experienced work environments where there is a hierarchy in which Black women are less likely to advocate for themselves or their needs. We are more likely to automatically assume a role of subservience. While our colleagues may have been raised to practice using their personal agency, we were not. As children, many of us were taught both explicitly and implicitly that we were meant to be seen and not heard and that we should not question those in authority. Since the time of slavery, these messages were meant to keep us safe, but they are no longer helpful in contemporary work environments. We need to actively unlearn those messages we received in childhood in order to learn to set boundaries, speak our truths, and know our worth in adulthood. Given that we were never taught these tools and that the opposite messaging has been ingrained in us for hundreds of years, no wonder this particular unlearning can be so difficult for us. Long-held societal structures continue to prevent Black women from advancing and experiencing true equality. We are paid less than our peers despite making up the demographic with the most advanced degrees,[1] our businesses and nonprofits receive less investment and philanthropic funding despite outperforming in the market with a fraction of the resources,[2] and our health complaints are not taken seriously, making us more susceptible to misdiagnoses, fatalities from preventable diseases and childbirth, and poor access to preventive care regardless of our education or class.[3]

What happens when we do take up more space in the world and advocate for ourselves? Although it can feel uncomfortable at first and takes practice, it is important to lean on your truth and stop accepting what no longer serves you, no matter how that is received by others. Connecting with and trusting your body are essential to advocating for yourself in the doctor's office. If you are not taken seriously in your workplace and don't receive the

---

1   Courtney Connley, "Black Women with College Degrees Still Make Less Than White Men Without," Chief, July 26, 2023, https://chief.com/articles/black-women -with-higher-education-still-make-less-than-white-men-without-degrees.

2   Nate Raymond, "Venture Capital Fund Defends Grants for Black Women in US Appeals Court," Reuters, January 31, 2024, www.reuters.com/sustainability/society -equity/venture-capital-fund-defends-grants-black-women-us-appeals-court -2024-01-31; Kimberly Pike, "Women of Color-Led Nonprofits Struggle for Survival Funding: Why?" *Philanthropy Women*, February 7, 2021, https://philanthropywomen .org/women-of-color/women-of-color-led-nonprofits-struggle-for-survival -funding-why.

3   Vidya Rao, "'You Are Not Listening to Me': Black Women on Pain and Implicit Bias in Medicine," Today, July 27, 2020, https://www.today.com/health/implicit-bias -medicine-how-it-hurts-black-women-t187866.

pay and title you deserve, practice advocating for yourself and recognize your value. Even if it takes time for the world to catch up to our practice of honoring our worth and see us as equals, we won't get in our own way. By advocating for ourselves, we'll standardize that behavior for the next generation. We understand and have compassion for our parents' and grandparents' generations, who exercised more limited agency out in the world because they were operating in a different context with different tools. While we still face some injustices similar to those they faced, we also have more access to tools to process information and gather and galvanize as a community. Although our liberties are constantly being threatened, the fact that we have them in the first place is because of our elders' sacrifices. We laud them for their sacrifices, even as we work toward greater progress and let go of practices that no longer serve us.

The strength of our community enables us to pick up the torch, build on the foundation of our predecessors, and press forward with both the lessons of the past and the sustenance of sustained hope. We lean on the legacy of our ancestors as we simultaneously make progress in how we show up in the world. I truly believe we sit in the crux of our ancestors' wildest dreams.

GO-DEEPER EXERCISE: REFRAMING
SELF-ADVOCACY

Take some time delving into the following reflection questions to identify areas in your life where you can begin advocating for your needs.

1. If you've experienced this, recall the first time you were not taken seriously in a medical setting. Jot down everything you remember and take note of any sensations that arise in your body as you recall that trauma. (If it begins to feel overwhelming, affirm those emotions and take a quick break to ground yourself in your breath if you need to.)

2. What workplace encounters have you had when your intelligence, experience, and/or position were undermined? What happened? If you did not stand up for yourself (perhaps to preserve your mental health and plan your exit), how did you respond in the moment? Reflecting on the tools presented in this book and any wisdom gained since that incident, how would you respond to that situation today? Spend some time visualizing this scenario with your ideal response.

3. Do you need to offer yourself forgiveness for not advocating for your best interests in the past? How can you reframe any negative beliefs about your abilities that arose from those incidents, recognizing that you didn't have the

knowledge you needed at the time to better navigate the situation?

4. When you were growing up, did you see Black women advocating for themselves? What messages did you receive, both explicitly and implicitly, based on what you witnessed?

5. Celebrate your progress by recalling instances when you saw growth in championing yourself over time.

BREATHWORK FOR SUSTAINING HOPE (ALTERNATE NOSTRIL BREATHING)

Maintaining a sense of hope out in the world can be difficult. As we are simultaneously navigating our own individual journeys while facing many obstacles being Black in the world, taking care to refill our cups is necessary in order to keep pressing forward. We can couple leaning in to our whys and being encouraged by the progress made by our elders with embodying a sense of hopefulness in our bodies with the breath. On the days when we are overwhelmed with the trauma all around us and the news cycle circulating images of Black bodies not honored with care, we will lean in to our tools in order to not succumb to hopelessness. Due to the number of steps in this particular breathwork pattern, alternate nostril breathing can be considered a more intermediate practice. If you are still working through feeling comfortable experimenting with different techniques of the breath, feel free to substitute for this pattern a more beginner-friendly practice, like the oceanic breath exercise shared in chapter 2.

1.   Start by making your physical space and body as comfortable as possible. (This practice is comfortable for most while done sitting up versus lying down.) Dim the lights and remove any distractions. Sinking into whatever surface is supporting you, close your eyes or gently gaze at an object in front of you or the tip of your nose.

2.   Raise the thumb and index finger of your preferred hand (or feel free to adjust this part to make it accessible to your abilities as long as you're able to touch your left and right nostrils). Note: The instructions below were written for the usage of your right hand. Reverse them for usage of your left.

3.   Plug your right nostril with your thumb, then inhale through the left nostril slowly, feeling your chest and diaphragm expand.

4.   Once you reach the top of the inhale, with lungs still full, release your right nostril and plug your left nostril with your index finger.

5.   Exhale out of the right nostril. Once lungs are depleted, inhale into the right nostril.

6.   Then plug the right nostril with your thumb. Exhale out of the left nostril.

7.   Continue the practice by inhaling into the left nostril before plugging it with your index finger and repeating the cycle of breaths. *(Hint: The nostril you exhale out of will be*

the same nostril you inhale into before plugging and exhaling out of the opposite nostril.)

8. Focus your attention on the air going into each nostril. Intentionally affirm your ability to find hope in the midst of despair out in the world into your own body and existence.

9. Get to know what your body needs with the amount of time you allocate to this practice. If you need only five minutes of practice time for this exercise, start with that. If you need a deeper practice in the future, set your timer for longer. Notice how your body feels with different intervals. Incorporate this exercise into your routine as needed.

Chapter 8

CRAFTING YOUR PERSONAL DEFINITION OF SUCCESS

WITNESSING OTHER PEOPLE live out their dreams on social media has, on one hand, given us a glimpse of realities that we hadn't even known were possible, but on the other hand, it has created a culture of comparison and envy. Content creators curate aspects of their lives to share on social media, giving viewers a warped perception of what their life is actually like. We don't see all their ups, downs, and behind-the-scenes realities of the lifestyle, career, or romantic relationship that appears perfect on their feed. Constantly comparing yourself to people that you do not really know sets you up for feeling like the life you've been dealt is a bad hand. Experiencing true contentment and fulfillment means honoring what a good life looks like for you, rather than what you see on Instagram or what others think your life should be. Understanding your motivations and values enough to create a life that feels good to you will be one of the most rewarding quests you can fulfill in your lifetime.

There is already a movement underway for Black women who are boldly and unashamedly redefining what life should look like on their own terms, regardless of cultural and familial ideals. Whether it comes to getting married and having kids later in life or opting out of climbing the corporate ladder to work independently, many of us are pursuing our own desires despite what others and even our past, unrealized selves have said. More and more of us are realizing how unfulfilling it is to pursue accolades that are not in alignment with our true desires.

ENSURE YOUR DREAMS ARE YOURS

As black girls breathing® has grown and received wider exposure, I am often approached by people who are inspired by my work and want to do something similar. When I follow up with a few questions, I often find that they don't actually want to put in the effort required of my career trajectory or fully understand the sacrifices I've made; they simply want to know what it feels like to achieve a certain level of success. They want to know what it feels like to be featured in top magazines and have work that impacts thousands. In reality, the press features are 2 percent of my overall workload, and when I initially started this company, I never imagined it would have this level of impact. There are so many sacrifices, obstacles, and nos involved in my profession that the people never see. We often don't see from afar what's required to achieve our dreams. Perhaps this is for the best, since we might not otherwise voluntarily sign up for all the losses, hard lessons, discipline, and long days and nights (that turn into years) required to reach our goals.

Your path may not look like mine or anyone else's, and it's not supposed to. All our journeys to achieve our dreams will have some bumps along the way, which makes it all the more important that you pursue what you truly want. Even after we've reached a goal, we continue to evolve and change and dream new dreams. It is essential that you give yourself the freedom to continuously explore, ask yourself the right questions, and rely on your internal resources to ensure that each step of your journey is right for you. Being honest with yourself will help you stay the course with confidence and self-trust as you build the right life for yourself.

GET TO THE ROOT OF YOUR DESIRES

One way to ensure you're not chasing dreams that aren't actually yours is to get to the root of your desires. Reflect on why you want something and where that desire comes from—whether it is intricately tied to an innate ambition or you believe it will give you a greater sense of purpose. You don't want to get lost spending a lifetime pursuing something that you never really wanted deep down. The reality is that your desires and your definitions of success will shift on many occasions over the course of your life. Doing the groundwork of thoroughly understanding your ambitions and desires while allowing yourself to evolve at any point in the process allows you to create a healthy balance between pursuing your dreams and also giving yourself space to grow, reevaluate, and make adjustments when necessary. We can stunt our own growth when we stifle our curiosity and close ourselves to unexpected opportunities because we're too focused on our original vision without allowing ourselves to evolve. As you reflect on some of your goals that embody your definition of success, ask yourself the following questions. Notice how your body responds and what, if any, emotions arise as you contemplate these questions.

EXPLORING THE ROOT OF YOUR DESIRES

- *Where did your vision of success originate?*
- *Who do you hope to become when you reach this level of success?*
- *Why do you think this particular goal will make you successful?*
- *Where did you get the idea that this goal would make you successful?*
- *Did your dream originate from a natural ability? Were you always told that you were great at something and that you should invest in this gift?*
- *Do you feel that accomplishing your goals will make you or other people proud?*
- *Do you feel a sense of obligation or joy when you reflect on this ambition?*
- *Are you inspired by anyone who has accomplished some aspect of this dream?*
- *Do you feel innate motivation to take steps toward this dream?*
- *If you don't accomplish this dream, what do you think will happen? What do you think this would say about you?*

These questions will help you explore the foundation of your desires and what an ideal life looks like to you. We want to be deeply in tune with our own desires and envision a life that isn't rooted in comparison.

After doing the work of examining the origins of your desires, you will go through several phases on the journey toward realizing your dreams: idealization, taking steps toward your destination, and evaluating the promised land. As ever-evolving human beings, it's important we allow our definitions of success to evolve with us.

IDEALIZATION: DEFINING THE "IDEAL" YOU

In my opinion, the idealization stage is one of the most exciting aspects of concocting a vision. At this stage, you're filled with positive feelings as you dream up possibilities for the future. Your imagination runs wild. You feel unstoppable and draw inspiration from others' stories of triumph. You notice how your past experiences, whether good or bad, led you to this moment when you are clear on what you want for your future. At this moment in time, you are fully focused on your ideal life. You're motivated to obtain the education you need to get closer to that dream. You feel comfortable making both temporary and long-term sacrifices to get there. At this point in your journey, optimism is high, you haven't experienced any struggles or bumps in the road, and the dream is pure and untainted by external realities or fear of failure. This stage is critical, so immerse yourself fully in the idealization process without jumping to potential pitfalls. Becoming too preoccupied with practical details at this early stage can sap all the energy you need to accomplish your dreams and make you wonder, *Why bother?* Allowing ourselves as Black women to get lost in the possibilities of life, to dream beyond what we've ever witnessed in our own families and communities growing up, is an act of resistance.

As we allow ourselves to think outside the box and refuse to be limited by the restrictions and negative perceptions placed upon us, we find a world of possibilities that rivals our ancestors' wildest dreams. Many of us have been conditioned to be alert to the harsh realities of the world, making it harder for us to dream—so there may be a lot of unlearning we need to do. And that's okay. The goal is for us to push past societal and familial norms that keep us small and limit our potential. We deserve to dream big and define what *big* means for ourselves. *Big* doesn't have to mean wearing designer brands or climbing the corporate ladder. For some, *big* might mean living an expansive life of ease that gives you plenty of time to rest. Your nervous system operates in a grounded state rather than fight-or-flight mode. You're able to spend more time with family and friends during the week and not just on the weekend. You have enough room in your schedule to attend every recital, game, or spelling competition that your child, niece or nephew, or mentee in your community puts on your calendar. There are endless possibilities for what a big or fulfilling life can look like. The goal is to always prioritize what's fulfilling to you and *only* you and to get as clear as possible on what that looks and feels like.

Being able to identify your desires and personal definitions of success starts with understanding how you'd like to *feel* as you navigate life. Because truth be told, in all that we do, we're not actually chasing the destination, the reward, the salary, or the position we're after. We're chasing a desired feeling that we think we'll experience once we've reached that goal. The breathwork and reflection exercises in this book are designed to help you identify how emotions show up in your body and better connect with how you feel. (Granted, I know that many of us have been conditioned to disconnect from our feelings, so the work described in this book requires continual unlearning. But don't forget to celebrate how far you've come as you get more comfortable discovering more about yourself.)

Prior to starting black girls breathing,® I founded two other companies. The first was a marketing consultancy serving small and midsized businesses, which I launched after leaving the global consumer goods marketing position in NYC. The consultancy met my definition of success at the time, as it allowed me to maintain the same lifestyle with a similar gross pay, minus the NYC living expenses, as my corporate job had. I went on to launch a second company, which, for lack of a better word, "failed." I put "failed" in quotation marks because that's how the outside world would describe having to shut down a business. But after the initial pain of closing its virtual doors subsided, I realized that my experience at that second company gave me the connections and deeper insight I needed to do business with large corporations when I started black girls breathing.® BGB would represent my most successful venture to date. The company has reached heights I never would have dreamed of while fulfilling my passion for seeing Black women live free of the strongholds of crippling, long-term trauma. While I never could have predicted how this journey would unfold (there's beauty in being openhanded with your vision and making space for the unexpected to happen), I've always been clear on what success would feel like. Those feelings have been my guiding light and compass. I've relied on that innate wisdom to decide which opportunities to decline, which to put on hold, and which to respond to with a clear, emphatic *Yes!* When the way forward has gotten murky, when unexpected trials and tribulations came my way, and even when I lost sight of the end goal because the current reality was overwhelming, somehow, I was able to refocus on my personal purpose and my definitions of success to redirect my path and evaluate whether I needed to change my route to my final destination.

Your Ideal Life

Whether it comes to how and where you'd like to wake up in the morning or how you like to relax, getting as specific as possible on what your ideal life would look like and how it would make you feel offers valuable information on your journey, helping you to keep going, course correct when necessary, and stay as aligned as possible with your definition of success as it evolves. An ideal day multiplied over and over (with the occasional, inevitable bad day thrown into the mix) creates ideal months and years that lead to an ideal life. So, let's get into the specifics of our days, using our five senses to guide us.

Close your eyes and envision what an ideal day would look like to you if there were no restrictions or barriers—from the moment you open your eyes in the morning to when you climb back into your bed at night. Nothing is off-limits. Use the following table to help you map out how your personal ideals translate into daily actions and habits. Return to these ideals as your internal compass to gauge whether your current habits are aligning or causing friction with your long-term goals. I've included some examples in the chart to help you craft your version(s) of an ideal day. Keep in mind it's your life, sis! You make the rules. Know that you can complete this exercise with your current season of life in mind and return to the chart to tweak it as you gather more information on what works for you and what doesn't.

Times of Day	Smell	See	Taste	Touch	Hear
In my ideal morning, I...		The sun rise and have time to journal when I wake up two hours before my day's activities begin (work, getting the kids ready for school, etc.). My mornings feel full of ease as I prioritize myself and my reflection time before doing anything for others. I don't have any screen time at this point.			

Times of Day	Smell	See	Taste	Touch	Hear
In my ideal afternoon, I...				My best friend's hand as I make time for sisterhood catch-ups and hangouts at least twice a month. Making time for community, no matter what is on my to-do list, makes me feel fulfilled, like the best version of myself.	The satisfaction of my clients in response to the projects I just finished on their behalf, which are completely aligned with my talents and gifts.
In my ideal evening, I...	A home-cooked dinner incorporating some of the current season's produce that I picked up from my local farmer's market or my own garden that I started the year before.				

Take it a step further and see how these daily actions have an impact on how your days, weeks, and months generally feel. And please note, I'm not asking you to bypass all the hard moments that you may encounter. In fact, this exercise is a great way to help you visualize how to take care of yourself when you have less-than-ideal days. Be gentle with yourself when you have difficult days.

Daily Behaviors I Implemented to Create an Ideal Week:
(Examples: Spending Sunday grocery shopping and meal planning/prepping to minimize cooking time during the week; incorporating a daily movement plan, like walking x amount of steps to relieve physical stress and increase energy levels throughout the day.)

_____

_____

_____

Weekly Behaviors and Routines That Created an Ideal Month:
(Example: Less time spent cooking during the week allowed me to cultivate joy and a sense of belonging by spending more time on hobbies and with my community.)

_____

_____

_____

Monthly, Quarterly, or Seasonal Behaviors and Routines That Created an Ideal Year:

(Example: Advance planning and being consistent with routines created a habit that allowed me to consistently invest in my areas of curiosity. I discovered a new career to explore, deep-dived into creative interests, or was able to reserve time to take a sabbatical for deep rest, all qualities that depict the type of lifestyle I wish to have and who I want to be in the world.)

_____

_____

_____

THE IN-BETWEEN STAGE: TAKING STEPS TOWARD YOUR DESTINATION

Navigating the "in-between" space toward our goals is uncomfortable for most people. I have yet to meet anyone who enjoys the process of not knowing whether their efforts will come to fruition. Our bodies experience a visceral reaction to leaving comfort and stability behind to trek toward the unknown, making us wonder at times why we decided to make this journey in the first place. Uncertainty disrupts our sense of safety and our desire for predictability. The reality is that once you leave the idealization stage, fueled by excitement and energy around what's to come, you will be tested in the in-between stage before you reach your goals. Various challenges will arise, which is a normal part of every journey, but they will make you question whether your ideal life is possible or worth weathering the storms and disappointments required to get there. Everyone's in-between stage will look different depending on their specific situation. Some of our greatest heroes have weathered many trials to get to where they are, but they were faithful in showing up for their dreams and desires day in and day out.

I've learned from my own experience that persistence and resilience are what take you to your goal. The road to get there will truly strengthen your sense of self, and you'll have plenty of opportunities to use your internal compass as you return to your whys with each obstacle you encounter. You'll need that personal conviction when your journey calls for sacrifice, self-belief (especially if there aren't a lot of people who support your ambitions or believe you can do it), and faith to keep going. You'll need to come face-to-face with your fears and dig into your mental and emotional toolbox to help you counter those urges to quit. And please know, sis, sometimes quitting is the best thing we can do for our long-term journeys. Remember how I shared earlier in this chapter about the failure of my second business? Well, though the "how" to realize my ideal life shifted, my fundamental desires and definitions of success stayed the same. Dissolving my second company gave me the learnings and connections I needed to make black girls breathing® a success. So know that stopping something and starting again, or trekking along a different path en route to your final destination, is not only possible but encouraged when you evaluate (more on this in the next section) new discoveries on your journey toward your goal. If your efforts aren't fruitful, use that information to course correct. Think about it. Your favorite apps and technological tools constantly have updates. Your favorite companies rebrand, add new product lines, and enter new markets that help them reach their overarching goals. So why can't you?

Demystifying the journey to achieve your dream life means preparing as much as possible ahead of time for the many occasions when you'll wonder why you're doing this brave, new thing to begin with. You may ask yourself, *Who do you think you are to even pursue this thing?* You may have to endure long stretches of your journey when there's only silence and the feeling of walking through a dark tunnel. You know your destination will be well lit, but in the meantime, you have to walk along an undefined and dark path to get there. It's par for the course, so equip yourself with the tools and understanding needed for the in-between stage now to avoid being blindsided later. Yes, you may still encounter unexpected challenges, but know that just because you encounter these roadblocks doesn't mean you're on the wrong path or that your desires aren't worth pursuing.

What are some tools you've picked up in this book that you can tap in to when you navigate fears and uncertainty during this in-between phase filled with unpredictability? How can you cultivate a safe, internal space to remind yourself of your end goal when you can take only one step at a time?

IS THIS WHAT I REALLY WANT? EVALUATING THE PROMISED LAND ONCE YOU ARRIVE

Although we don't often hear our heroes talk about this, it isn't uncommon to reach a long-sought-after goal only to feel underwhelmed by the result. Deciding that a former dream looks and feels different than you expected once you arrive is perfectly okay. In fact, it's an integral part of our life journey as we get clear on what our desires are and what fulfillment looks like to us. Sometimes it takes getting a thing we thought we wanted to realize that the pursuit made it shinier and more desirable than it actually was. Or sometimes we do enjoy the fruits of our labor but it's short-lived; we might get more out of the journey than the destination because it's a testament to our perseverance and mental, emotional, and physical endurance, which further builds our self-trust and self-esteem. The accomplishment fuels our confidence in our abilities. Although your destination may look and feel different than you first imagined, what you learned along the way still makes it a rich experience. Your ability to have a flexible mindset around any perceived misstep will help you make the necessary adjustments to your dream or dream a new dream altogether.

Once you've achieved your goal, it's important that you own your experience of it. Perhaps there are a lot of other people who would love to be in your shoes and imagine your experience to feel a certain way. As a result, you may feel guilty that what you, too, thought would be a fulfilling experience ended up feeling somewhat anticlimactic. I want to normalize that realization. You can be grateful for your experience and still be honest if it looks different from what you expected. It is important to prioritize your own joy and your definitions of success, which takes practice in a world where many people feel burdened by ideas of what they "should" do with their lives. Each individual's culture, education, socioeconomic background, and personal feelings and inclinations influence what they think is possible for their lives and can create internal barriers that prevent them from moving on from old dreams to new ones as they dare to dream bigger.

Maybe someone's childhood dream was to become a doctor. They passionately pursued the education they needed to make this dream a reality while receiving encouragement from their community that had never seen a doctor that looked like them. After this person got their white coat and had been practicing medicine for a while, they decided to take what they had learned and become a professor. It was a hard choice for them to make because they felt they were letting their family and community down, but they could no longer ignore the thirst they had to try something new. It can be difficult to make changes like these because of others' attachment to the old dream and all the challenges that come with starting over. It's common to assess our happiness and sense of success through the lens of others' perceptions, and it can feel costly to lose their esteem by leaving behind one achievement in pursuit of another. But you can trust your inner compass to help you decide whether or when to redefine your dreams at any point.

THE INNER RUMBLINGS OF A SHIFT

Rarely does anyone wake up one day and decide to make a drastic change in their life. More often than not, I've found that when someone is ready to move on to another chapter in their life, the signs begin to show up gradually. You start feeling restless, curious, or even bored. Along with that urge to make a change, guilt may arise, leading to an inner dialogue that might sound something like *I should be grateful for what I have now. Who am I to want more?* While society might inflict that guilt upon us, it's possible to be both grateful and hopeful for more—we're allowed to feel and honor more than one emotion at the same time. Even if you're not 100 percent ready to commit to a new thing, allow yourself to follow the breadcrumbs of curiosity, so to speak. This will gradually guide you to any number of possibilities for your next chapter.

GO-DEEPER EXERCISE: FOLLOW THE BREADCRUMBS

Whether you're on the cusp of a breakthrough or just trying to see what else life can offer, you can likely find clues all around you that provide insight into your ideal next steps. I call this exercise "follow the breadcrumbs" because we tend to overlook small but important details in our lives. Find a quiet place and grab a warm or cold drink—whatever suits your fancy. Turn on a calming playlist to really set the mood for self-exploration. Honor and refrain from judging whatever responses first come to mind. There are no wrong answers—these are simply starting points for deeper reflection around potential changes you'd like to make.

Deepening Your Natural Abilities

The people closest to me come to me for _____

_____.

I'm always receiving compliments on how well I_____

_____.

What is something(s) that doesn't require much time or effort for me to do but seems harder for other people?

Following Your Curiosity

I'm interested in learning about _____

_____.

The last time I got really excited about something was _____

_____.

If I were able to change anything for a day, I would: _____

_____.

Closing Out a Chapter

_____ used to feel fulfilling or exciting but no longer does.

The time I've invested in _____ makes me hesitant to abandon it because I don't want to feel like I've wasted my time.

I feel obligated to do _____ because of what other people think.

Chapter 9

MAKING PEACE WITH FAILURE

ON YOUR JOURNEY toward healing and thriving, you'll encounter many detours along the way. The roadblock that seems to cause many people the most mental and emotional stagnation is failure. *Failure* is such a loaded term that tends to invoke deep shame and regret. The very thought of something not going exactly as planned can deter you from even trying to take another step or begin a new chapter, but a life well lived requires us to repeat the cycle of trying and potentially failing many times. Stopping ourselves before we even start to explore new opportunities, take it up another notch, or reconfigure our lives because of the fear of failure holds so many of us back from seeing our true potential or discovering different facets of ourselves. What would your life look and feel like if you were able to see failure less like a source of doom and more like an opportunity to be curious and open and gather information for your next best step? And furthermore, how much lighter would you feel if you were able to release the guilt of all the perceived failures of your past? Getting to that place requires some deep reflection about the beliefs and stories we're telling ourselves about failure. A life fully lived is one driven more by faith and curiosity and less by our fears of negative and unplanned outcomes because we know that disappointments do not affect our inherent value or how we can best navigate the world.

I've encountered many Black women in their fifties and older in our black girls breathing® community who have shared their journeys and imparted wisdom to the younger women in our sessions. They have often shared about their need to work through past regrets that were exacerbated by others' judgments, the difficulty of recognizing failure as a normal life experience rather than a sign of personal shortcomings, and how they were using the present moment and their newfound self-awareness to make braver choices. Being haunted by dreams that they never explored and what feels like decades of lost time has led them to the point where they prefer confronting their fears to being stuck in inaction. Decades of life experience has taught them not to worry about other people's opinions. They warn younger generations that others' opinions are ultimately not worth the sacrifice, telling them, "Don't be like me." Don't let our elders' experiences be in vain. Let's learn to reframe failure as a powerful tool to live a fulfilling life.

EMBRACING THE UNKNOWN

The ideal life that you began to map out in the previous chapter can happen for you. The magic and miracle of that journey is not knowing all the details yet. While you can't plan all the details of your future, you can be confident in your ability to navigate in the unknown. You don't know what challenges will surface that, if alchemized, can accelerate your journey even further. You don't know ahead of time what heartbreaks, betrayals, and hard lessons may happen along the way. These are the parts of the journey that no one really wants to talk about or even imagine when they're envisioning a beautiful future, especially if they've already experienced many hardships just to get to a place where they can begin to dream again. I truly wish I could tell you that after you address your individual and generational traumas and learn to better manage your stress, the rest of your life will be all flowers and sunshine. But unfortunately, that's not the reality. There's a normal human tendency to want to be done dealing with hard things, especially if we've already been courageous enough to confront all the hard things of the past. And since we, Black women in particular, experience deep-seated perfectionism, we may think that once we've identified the unhealthy patterns of our pasts, we just need to be hypervigilant to avoid experiencing anything similar in the future. But constantly being on our guard is exhausting and unsustainable. Trying to map out all the details of our lives to avoid potential pitfalls can give us a false sense of security. While we may *feel* in control, we can't actually anticipate every challenge that may come our way, and sis, that's just too much work to try to prepare for the next phase of your life. It's better to direct your energy toward dropping the protective guards that aren't actually serving you, while maintaining whatever boundaries you need and opening your hands to receive all that life has for you.

Your journey will include many twists and turns, but trusting yourself to use your tools to get through them will be your super-power. Giving yourself grace as you take risks, try new things, and explore all that life has to offer while allowing yourself to make mistakes and learn from them will give you a more robust life than being overly cautionary ever will. And I understand the fears that we're up against. Our ancestors experienced real threats when they took the slightest risk, and we've inherited that trauma in our bodies. This fear has been reinforced in our own experiences with society as well. While one mistake might have cost our ancestors their lives, a fact that cannot be bypassed, we also recognize the shifts in society that have given us greater freedom than our predecessors had (and please note I am by no means denying the problems that still exist today). We now get the opportunity to choose a new way of operating and responding to the world around us.

Think of a past situation when you've "failed." What emotions immediately rise up in your body and where? Set a timer for fifteen minutes and allow yourself to freewrite and emote on paper. When you've finished verbalizing your experience, check in with the body part(s) where you felt the emotions. Set another timer for five minutes (or more if your body needs it) to make space for these emotions to rise up in the body with the breathwork practice in the "Go-Deeper Exercise" section at the end of this chapter. Keep affirming yourself, even if the emotions are difficult. You are right where you need to be.

DECENTERING OTHERS' OPINIONS

If we are being honest with ourselves, at the core of our fear of failure are not just our personal beliefs but the looming question of *How will others view me?* The "others" we're most concerned about are often those closest to us. These might be parental figures or the people who have had front-row seats for a large portion of our lives and have had time to form opinions of us, creating neat, little boxes in which they think we should fit. It's not intentional that they construct such rigid definitions of who we are and who we could become, but it's human nature to expect people to behave the way we've always seen (or perceived) them to behave in the past. Our awareness of others' expectations can add to our own fear of change when we're contemplating a shift in life where failure is a possibility. Taking others' perceptions of you into account can be healthy. There's a system of checks and balances in place when those who care about you offer advice and guidance that give you a more well-rounded perspective on your situation and potential blind spots. However, this system gets out of balance when you put more weight on outside opinions than your own instincts. Since Black women are conditioned to care too much about how others perceive us, the way we view ourselves is often too heavily dependent on external factors, including others' opinions, perspectives in the media, and popular trends. The more we can center our own values and perspectives of ourselves, the less disoriented we'll feel when things don't go according to plan or we need to take a different route in life. We'll make decisions with our best interests in mind, instead of delaying our long-term happiness because we are overly concerned about how others will perceive our decisions and changes in behavior.

After I experienced early success in New York—working an intense corporate job, which made it possible for me to rent my own one-bedroom apartment at the age of twenty-two—I made some big life changes that made me feel like a failure at the time. While living in New York, I'd been dating someone long-distance for a year and a half. I was burned out from my job, so I decided to start my first company and move to Tennessee to cultivate that relationship despite my parents' reservations. I convinced them that it was a good, well-thought-out decision. (Well, I sort of told them after I made the decision.) Long story short, that relationship ended up being a toxic and draining situation; we split up, and I moved back to my mom's house in Atlanta. I felt so ashamed that I needed the emotional and financial safety net of returning home to heal from a traumatic breakup and rebuild my life. I thought, *If only I had listened to my mother, I wouldn't be in this situation. I wouldn't need to rebuild my life from scratch after all I worked so hard to achieve in New York.*

At this point, I had started working on my second business (that, as you know, ended up failing), and I was struggling mentally and emotionally. My sense of self-worth had taken a huge hit, and word of my breakup and departure from Tennessee had spread among my friends and past clients there. In order not to succumb to despair, I had to promise myself that I would center myself and my beliefs, rather than allow others' perceptions of my situation to dominate my thoughts. I had to process my guilt and shame while also affirming the younger version of me who had made the best decisions she could with the information she had at the time. Had I been naive to move in with someone that I hadn't truly known while dating long-distance? Yes. Was I the first twentysomething to get swept off her feet by charm and love bombing? No. Would I be the last? Absolutely not. Did I make the most of the situation by starting my own company and seeing how I was able to create something and excel at it? Yes. Did that first venture give me the courage to start another one? Yes. And when that second venture failed, did I have the confidence to try again? Yes. Did processing my emotions and learning to trust myself more than the opinions of others help me to heal my trauma and start afresh when it felt like my life had crumbled around me? Yes.

Looking at the situation as a whole helped me to focus on the present moment and make the shifts I needed for my next chapter in life, while I also extended grace to the younger version of myself who had made some mistakes. I hadn't been able to see past the fairy tale and the false promises I'd been sold, but I ultimately learned some valuable lessons from that experience.

EXERCISE TO DECENTER OTHERS' OPINIONS AND PRIORITIZE YOUR NEEDS

Close your eyes and reflect on the opinions that others have of you that are causing you to hesitate or making you feel judged or ashamed. Whose voices are those? Do these voices actually carry weight in your life? Why or why not? Jot down the responses that first come to mind to help identify any external opinions where you can begin to shift your focus to your own needs.

RESHAPING YOUR NARRATIVE

Can you relate to my story? Have you experienced failure or disappointment when things didn't turn out the way you expected, and yet you still survived? Or better yet, did you learn how to thrive? Resist the lie that you are a failure and can never do anything right. You dared to step outside the box and explore new possibilities for what your life could look like despite the risks and uncertainty. Do you feel like you've fallen behind or that you're not as successful as your peers? Know that you have a unique path, and comparison will only prevent you from fulfilling your own destiny. We have to be honest about our thoughts and feelings in the aftermath of failure or disappointment so we can process perceived missteps and move forward. Anyone who has combatted negative thought patterns or beliefs understands how much energy it takes to get out of that cycle. While we may continue to experience fear and self-doubt, we can live courageously. We exercise self-compassion and validate our feelings by speaking directly to those thoughts and calming our fears.

I want to be transparent that challenging feelings of failure can be triggering. Often, these fear-based narratives have a stronghold on our beliefs about ourselves, so confronting these negative thoughts can trigger an identity crisis. For example, you may have a friend who self-identifies as having an anxious personality. Even if she's been clinically diagnosed with anxiety, that diagnosis isn't her whole identity. Yet she may have a hard time separating her anxiety from how she sees herself and what she can accomplish; she might center her anxiety when it comes to how she shows up in life. It's the difference between saying, "I'm an anxious person" and "I experience anxiety." While the former feels like an all-encompassing identity, the latter phrase gives us permission and space to not project anxiety onto every situation we encounter; we might actually surprise ourselves with our courage to show up in new chapters of life in different capacities in spite of our diagnoses. Acknowledging a reality while not giving it all of our agency is empowering. While your friend may have had experiences when she felt like her anxiety inhibited her, who she is and how she will show up in the future don't have to be dictated by her past. She does not have to impose an anxious identity on herself, because she is so much more than her anxiety. If she's used to projecting her anxiety onto every new situation, she may experience resistance around trying to separate anxiety from her identity at first. Why? Because we've used certain beliefs and narratives to keep us safe as we navigate the uncertainties of life. Our personal narratives act as a security blanket, and boy do we use them. However, there are so many more possibilities in life when we detach ourselves from limited narratives. (And please note I am in no way downplaying the severity of living with anxiety. As someone who's navigating an autoimmune condition, I've used this framework to not define myself solely by that reality.)

As we rewrite our narratives about past failures and perceived limitations, we can allow our bodies to fully feel the emotions associated with those experiences while not letting those emotions define our narratives. For example, you might experience the feeling of extreme disappointment and shame as a sensation of your heart sinking to the pit of your stomach. Connecting with the emotion and where it is showing up in your body will allow you to fully address that fear, observe the beliefs that arise from it, and counteract those beliefs with your current reality. Use the following table to deep-dive into specific emotions related to the fear of failure that surfaced for you as you read.

The Emotion I'm Feeling	The Place in My Body Where I Feel the Emotion	The Beliefs Arising from That Emotion	My Current Reality
Shame, unworthiness	My heart space / chest area	I'm so stupid for making that decision. I'll never be able to recover from that. I wish I could go back in time.	Although things didn't pan out how I wanted, I've learned so much from past mistakes. I've demonstrated that I can trust myself more moving forward and have all that I need to tackle what life may bring my way.

WHAT'S THE WORST THAT COULD HAPPEN?

When it comes to facing my fear of failure, sometimes I let my mind "go there" all the way. As I've worked to reshape the long-standing narratives and beliefs that have fueled some of my behavioral patterns, I've found that accepting those thoughts as they arise (rather than condemning myself for feeling those things in the first place) releases a lot of anxiety and pressure. As a former self-work addict (I've since decided I don't always need to feel like I'm "working on myself") who is totally committed to the healing process, let me paint a picture for you. A negative thought or belief keeps arising in mind. Before I can even observe the thought and reshape the belief, I experience self-judgment because the thought has come up in the first place and I need to do the self-work to address it. So, on top of whatever anxiety this thought has caused, I now experience even greater stress about feeling stressed. Can you see how that has a compounding effect? As someone who's seen as an expert at helping others process their stress, I experience thoughts like *Now, girl, how are you leading others if you're still working through your own stress?* You've likely experienced similar self-condemnation as you've done your own inner work. I've learned to respond to thoughts like these by accepting that they will inevitably come up, while also challenging them by following them to their fearful conclusions. I'm careful to engage in this activity when I have the mental and emotional capacity to feel the triggers while still being grounded in my body. If a thought feels like it might trigger a negative spiral, I tap in to some breathwork or do some active meditation while walking to help ground me so I can explore that thought in depth at a later time. It's important to go at your pace when you're feeling triggered. When I'm feeling grounded enough to engage with "worst-case scenario" thoughts, I follow those thoughts to see where they lead me. This exercise allows me to accept whatever part of me is trying to keep me "safe" while also responding to that fear in a productive way that actually moves me forward.

What does that actually look like? The following is an example of how I might engage with a doomsday thought like *What if you put out this product and no one uses it, or it gets tons of negative feedback?* I tap deeper in to that thought with an *Okay, then what?*

> **Fearful thought:** *And then you don't reach your goal, and everyone will consider you a failure.*
>
> **Me:** *Okay, I see your concern. Then what? What else would happen?*
>
> **Fearful thought:** *You'd be proving all your critics right. You weren't able to do it. It was too big of a goal.*
>
> **Me:** *Okay, I hear you. What do you think you're trying to protect me from?*
>
> **Fearful thought:** *Ruining all you've already created and becoming a laughingstock. I'm trying to protect you from ruining your self-esteem and your life.*
>
> **Me:** *Okay, wow. That is a big fear. I understand your concern. Is there another time you felt this way?*
>
> **Fearful thought:** *Yeah, it is a big risk. Remember those times in the past when you tried and it didn't work out? Remember how you felt afterward?*
>
> **Me:** *You mean the time I started a new business and it didn't work out? I do remember. I was pretty devastated and struggled with a lot of self-doubt as a result.*

Fearful thought: *Exactly. I don't want you to relive that experience ever again. I'm warning you for your own good.*

Me: *I hear you. That was hard, but do you remember what happened after that? I was able to take those learnings and apply them in the next chapter. I'd made all these great connections that were useful for the next business, and I was able to use all of my gifts and capabilities in ways that I hadn't imagined before, even though my original business idea didn't work out.*

Fearful thought: *That's true. But what if things don't work out as well as that time?*

Me: *Well, that's a possibility. But what if it does work out? There's a fifty-fifty chance. And if the fear is that people won't like the product, maybe we can try it out with a smaller group of people first to get their reactions and gather feedback before sharing it with a larger group. That may improve our chances of success.*

Fearful thought: *That's a good idea.*

Me: *I think so, too. That'd be a great next first step to address some of your concerns. Let's take it one day at a time. I appreciate you for bringing up this concern. I'll continue to listen to what you have to say so we can strategize.*

Fearful thought: *You're welcome. And I appreciate you listening. I don't mean to stress you out. I'm just trying to do my job and keep you safe.*

> **Me:** *I know. But I also know that I'm no longer the twenty-five-year-old who made those mistakes. I'm older now and have learned so much since then. We've been through a lot together; we've been able to navigate unexpected challenges and get to the other side. I trust us a bit more now. We have the tools we need to deal with the unexpected.*
>
> **Fearful thought:** *You're right. Thanks for seeing me. Thanks again for listening.*

By allowing my mind to go there with those thoughts, while staying present in my body and feeling the emotions and concerns as they arise, I am able to neutralize my worry about future scenarios that I can't possibly predict. I make space to express my fears while coming up with practical next steps to address those fears. It is empowering to face our fears head-on rather than try to suppress them. By allowing our fears to be felt, heard, and seen and addressing those concerns, we defuse the situation before the fear can escalate to worsening symptoms meant to get our attention, like aches, uneasiness, and ruminating over debilitating thoughts.

Although we're sometimes told to be fearless, the truth is that in facing the unknown, sometimes our fears do become a reality. Our fears aren't just figments of our imagination. Rather, our fears often carry an element of truth to them when we think about our histories and how some of our fears have come to pass. The imprint of that experience on our minds and bodies is very real. Rather than gaslighting ourselves, we can acknowledge those legitimate fears. We can compassionately listen to them, use the lessons of the past to avoid making the same mistakes, and explore the worst-case scenario to inspire new solutions.

GO-DEEPER EXERCISES: WORST-CASE SCENARIO SCRIPTING

As demonstrated in the "What's the Worst That Could Happen?" section, allowing your mind to follow the depths of a fear can reduce the paralyzing hold it can have on you. "Hearing out" the concerns, no matter how irrational, and addressing them directly can help the nagging to subside. As the intention for many of your fears is to "keep you safe," exploring the fear and following where it wants to take you can also provide you with insights on ways to better prepare for the journey that you're about to take. Use the script format outlined in the previous section to follow a major recurring fear down the rabbit hole, addressing each objection that arises with *Okay, then what?* to explore it fully. At the end of the exercise, take note of any insight that surfaces for you that will be helpful in preparing for the next step in your journey.

BREATHWORK FOR SELF-ACCEPTANCE AND FORGIVING PERCEIVED FAILURES: THREE-PART BREATH (ONE INHALE, TWO EXHALES)

You are more than how others have experienced you. You are even more than the limitations you may have placed on yourself. Let's give you an opportunity to envision and feel the expansiveness of your body with the breath. Reflect back on your responses in the activity earlier in this chapter about any emotions you experience around failure (on page 180). We'll use the following breathwork practice to be intentional about bringing awareness to that area and shifting any stagnant energy and emotion that live there.

1.   Lying down (or in whatever position feels accessible to you), check in with your body.

2.   Think about an experience of failure. Where do you feel it in your body? (If you're not completely sure or you can't identify a specific body part that feels this emotion, do a gentle scan to check in with each area of the body. Does your throat feel scratchy or like you can't swallow? Does your chest feel tight? Is your stomach queasy? Do your arms feel stiff or tingly? Does your heart feel raw or extremely exposed?) If a specific area feels vulnerable or in need of comfort, gently give it love with a nurturing touch. You can massage this area in a circular motion, first going clockwise, then counterclockwise.

3.   We'll further strengthen the mind-body connection by doing a one-part-inhale, two-part-exhale breathwork sequence: Opening your mouth as wide as possible, inhale into it, then exhale out of it once, halfway emptying your lungs. Then with another open-mouth exhale, empty the remaining air in your lungs. Try to connect your inhales and exhales so that when you feel your belly collapse from the last exhale, you immediately draw another breath for your open-mouth inhale. Elongating your breath, tune

in to your body as your stomach and chest rise with the inhale and deflate with the exhale. As you do this, envision the weight of the past failure melting from your body. With each inhale, breathe acceptance and self-compassion into your body. You truly did the best that you could, sis.

What have you noticed about your breath while progressing through the exercises in this book? Have you noticed any changes in how your breath sounds? Have your inhales and exhales deepened? Allow yourself to be curious and explore your body and its response to the breath as you continue to dive into these practices.

Chapter 10

THRIVING AND FREE

CLOSE YOUR EYES and tune in to all of your senses. Ask yourself, *What would it feel like in my body to be free?* Maybe your body would feel light. You would see nothing but future possibilities and your own resilience when you look in the mirror. You would have a strong sense of self. You would be able to show up for yourself in good times and challenging times, knowing that you have the tools to figure it out. You would trust yourself and your abilities, remembering all the past times you made it through as evidence that you can do that again and again, even during life's darkest seasons. You might feel some natural fear when you step out of your comfort zone, but you take whatever action is necessary to progress in spite of the fear. You know that you deserve to explore all the desires of your heart, so regardless of the risks, you leave no talent unused because the world truly, truly needs what you've got. As you reflect on how freedom would feel in your body and manifest outwardly in your life, you might wonder how you can find this level of freedom and why it matters so much for our community. We'll explore those questions in this chapter.

GENERATIONAL JOY AND INNER FREEDOM

We do our history an injustice by focusing only on generational trauma without the generational joy that is also part of our legacy. I see so much generational joy in my maternal grandmother and grandfather. At the time of this writing, my grandmother just celebrated her ninety-first birthday. She has witnessed deep, unconscionable traumas in the course of her life. Over the past few years that she's been living with and being taken care of by my mom, I've found myself making the thirty-five-minute drive to their house just to experience both her and my mom's maternal presence. I'm amazed by their innate joy and hope. It's a "no matter what" kind of hope born of witnessing some of the darkest atrocities in this country—from the effects of slavery to the persecution experienced during the civil rights movement. As my grandma would say in her Southern accent, she's seen "some thangs." Yet she still managed to be here.

And she doesn't simply exist, but she lives with a glimmer and twinkle in her eye and with old-time gospel hymns praising God's goodness still on her lips. On any given Sunday, after my grandmother has cycled through her favorite shows on MSNBC, you can hear her call out from her walker, "Hey, Google, play Mahalia Jackson." Tapping her knees with rheumatoid arthritic hands, she hums along to "How I Got Over" with a knowing vibrato. My grandmother isn't just observing Jackson's faith from a distance or admiring her sultry vocals. Oh, no—my grandmother has lived and attested to these lyrics. They've made way for an unshakable faith and innate joy. You'll hear my grandma say, "Oh, how I got over," and then belt out an old-time churchy affirmation: "This joy I have—the world didn't give it, and the world can't take it away."

This joy is a powerful tool. Just being in the presence of that joy during my lowest moments when I'm wondering why I'm doing this work fills my cup and reminds me of the steadfastness that runs in my DNA. After having discussed the effects of generational trauma and epigenetics in chapter 3, I'd be remiss to not discuss the importance of this infectious generational joy that is also part of our legacy. Gospel, blues, rock, and soul music manifest this generational joy. Our scientific inventions were created from this generational joy.

I have to believe that many of our abolitionists and civil rights activists found a deep well of strength in the idea that we, Black folks, deserve to experience even more joy in our current realities rather than just waiting for it in the afterlife because living in this world was so painful and unbearable. That hope for a future joy helped propel our predecessors forward in the darkest times to search for external freedom, in spite of the inherent dangers of that yearning.

I hope you, too, are inspired by our ancestors' fervor and cling to it in your own life as well. As I always mention in our black girls breathing® breathwork sessions and sunday balm® community, my intention is never to ignore the realities and the inherent dangers of occupying a Black body. The truth is that we don't yet have the privilege of experiencing full freedom. As I struggled with my own sense of hopelessness while consistently needing to fight and push against biases while doing this work, I found peace in my North Star: helping Black women cultivate a sense of inner freedom even while we have not fully experienced freedom in the world around us. It is my intention that in our ninety-minute sessions or however long we are in community together, each Black woman will experience what it's like to feel seen, heard, and witnessed in their vulnerabilities. As our ancestors have already shown us, inner freedom trumps the harsh realities of our existence and gives us something that's uniquely ours.

Making a home within your own body is a form of activism. While our capitalist society works overtime to ensure that there are still strongholds of all kinds preventing Black and Brown people from being free, we have an opportunity to ensure that this ideology doesn't seep into our bones. Cultivating a sense of autonomy and dignity in the midst of oppression has been our people's strength for centuries. While we work hard to dismantle systems that are actively trying to destroy us and rid us of all hope, our superpower lies in the belief that within our body, mind, and spirit, we can foster a freedom that this world cannot strip away from us. As we cling to our internal sense of freedom, we'll have the strength and fortitude to work for progress in the external world, one day at a time. So how do we nurture this internal sense of freedom and make our bodies a safe refuge from the outside world? We can start by making sure our own minds are a safe space to express our authenticity.

REWIRING NEGATIVE SELF-TALK

How do you speak to yourself on any given day? In the morning when you rise, are you gentle with yourself? What about when you make a perceived mistake? Are your thoughts harsh and punitive? How we view ourselves will be a litmus test for how we respond to the world around us and how the external world views us.

As you go about your day, notice the thoughts and narratives that most frequently cross your mind. If you notice any harsh words, trace them back to their origin. Has someone else said those things to you? Whose voice do you hear when it comes to those thoughts? Did those beliefs begin to take shape because of a specific event? One effective way to begin rewiring some of the harmful, subconscious thoughts that play on autopilot in your mind is to record affirmations via voice memo that you can listen to when you want to counteract your most common negative belief patterns. Hearing positive affirmations in your own voice can help you reframe repetitive, harmful thoughts and cultivate a friendship with yourself.

When you've worked through your own negative self-talk, it'll be easier to bypass others' unfounded critiques of you. As we work to rewire thoughts that might otherwise send us into a negative spiral, it's also important to not take every thought so seriously. Our minds are like sponges. We don't always know where we might have picked up an idea, and we do not need to attach ourselves to every single one. We can simply observe a thought with curiosity and emotional distance without overly identifying ourselves with it. As we learned in the chapter on generational trauma, those negative thoughts may not have originated with us or been a part of our own lived experience.

Mastering that cycle of negative thinking will be a critical first step in rewiring deeply embedded belief patterns that prevent you from even dreaming about an ideal life for yourself. You deserve to live to your full potential, sis.

REWIRING NEGATIVE THOUGHT PATTERNS

Negative Thought		Countering Affirmation
You can never get anything right.	→	I allow myself the space to be curious and try something new, knowing that when I start, I may not be an expert but I owe it to myself to try.
You should've known better. You shouldn't have made that mistake.	→	I'm not going to punish my younger self for not knowing what I now know. Because of what I've learned, I know how I'd like to show up in the future.
Why can't I be more like [insert name]?	→	I am unique, and so is my journey. I can't compare myself to someone whose life I don't know the full details of. I don't know their unique struggles and pain. I trust that my life will have its own wonders.

Use the blank spaces below to enter your own thoughts you're now ready to rewrite.

_____	→	_____
_____	→	_____
_____	→	_____
_____	→	_____

REDUCING YOUR PAIN TOLERANCE

When you begin to operate in a new way and stop seeing yourself solely through the lens of what you can do for others, you will carry a lighter load, thereby reducing your pain tolerance. And I deeply, deeply want more Black women to be able to tolerate less, especially when it comes to our relationships and our work in the world. Let's stop aiming to be a strong superwoman and just be human. A human who needs breaks and deserves to be seen, heard, and celebrated. A human who allows herself to try, make mistakes, and learn just like the rest of the world. Let's stop placing unnecessary expectations to be perfect on ourselves when humans are imperfect and can't know everything all the time. Although we've been conditioned for perfection, we can defy this conditioning. We can stop placing such heavy and unrealistic weights on our shoulders while not expecting that of others. Internalized racism is real. So if you're overloading yourself, you have normalized this behavior not just for you but for the other Black women in your life. After you do the individual work of releasing what you're not meant to carry, you'll also have to accept what it means for other

Black women in your life to stop doing so much. How will you support them in their journey instead of feeling inconvenienced?

Once you experience the benefits of centering yourself and shouldering less of the weight that, frankly, doesn't belong to you, it'll become easier to operate that way all the time. After you walk through the muck and discomfort that naturally come with shifting away from people-pleasing toward centering yourself, disappointing others by prioritizing yourself will no longer have as much of an effect on you as it may have had in the past. You'll be able to send a text declining an invitation or request without worrying so much about the other person's reaction. You'll begin to recognize the imbalance in certain relationships and do the work to find an equilibrium. And in the same vein, you won't peer pressure your sistah-friend to go beyond her limits but will be okay with being on the receiving end of a response like "I know I used to do that, but I can't any longer" or just a simple "No." You'll experience a new way of operating in the world that requires much less self-sacrifice and much more self-consideration.

You'll begin to get comfortable quitting things—often and fast. You'll no longer wait until a situation gets dire before recognizing that it's no longer serving you. You'll lean in to your intuition more often, using the tools offered in this book to develop a better relationship with your body so you listen to it and don't continuously push yourself beyond your capacity and to the point of disease. The voice of shame that would surface when you started standing up for yourself will begin to quiet. You may feel triggered at times by others' negative reactions, but you'll lean on the wisdom that those people's opinions won't matter that much to you in the long run. In short, "They'll be aight."

It's important to know that these new mindsets require unlearning old beliefs. As we've discussed, unlearning can come with periods of grief and discomfort before a sense of ease emerges after more practice. Although you'll be seeing yourself in a new light, you will still grieve for your former self and all that you might have lost in the past by not showing up in this way sooner. When that phase hits, it's important to practice deep compassion and kindness, not punish yourself for evolving and knowing better now than you did before.

Despite what mainstream wellness brands might say, the results may not be instantaneous. Unraveling years, decades, and generations of old thought patterns and behaviors may at times feel difficult, but I promise you this: it will be well worth the journey. And, sis, you are well on your way.

THE FEAR OF SUCCESS

Though we explored moving past the fear of failure in the previous chapter, the fear of success is on the other side of the coin. I want to first validate the deep, visceral fear that Black women feel when we put ourselves out there to be seen fully. For one thing, there have been few examples of Black women doing that without becoming a target that others—both within and outside our community—try to take down. The very act of taking up space and owning who we are elicits a response that many of us heard during our formative years when we were children exploring our identity: "Who do you think you are?" That question is always leveled with the intention of putting someone in their place and instilling self-doubt. When a seed of self-doubt is planted in a little Black girl, the idea that she internalizes well into her adulthood is simple: be small and invisible.

The accusation "Who do you think you are?" instills fear in so many of us—so much so that it prevents us from even trying to fulfill our personal definitions of success. We may do the arduous work of pushing past perceived limitations and allowing ourselves to dream about a life where we can be truer to ourselves. We may even make strides toward carrying out those dreams and get a taste of success. But often when we reach new heights, a fear of becoming too successful emerges. The novelty of things going well for you without the other shoe dropping can feel so unsettling. Throw into the mix new challenges like close friends not truly being happy for you, or having a harder time finding peers the higher you climb, or experiencing greater opposition as one of the few Black women at this level. But the most painful challenge may come from our own community when you reach new levels and they ask, "Who do you think you are?" This might be followed by another jealous remark: "You think you're all that." The crabs-in-a-barrel mentality stems from internalized racism. Therefore, it's hard to see one of us shining and doing well without thinking they're out of line. This reinforces the belief that people, especially people in our own community, want us to do well but not *too* well—not in a way that challenges their deep-seated beliefs about what's possible for a Black woman. Reaching new heights is beyond the scope of their imagination. Although this is a difficult reality to acknowledge, it reaffirms that the limitations we place on ourselves are a product of our environment. These limitations originated in the fields, where slave owners tried to extinguish our hope, cultures, identities, and pride. They accomplished part of their mission, but it's our job and our ancestors' dream to undo that damage and reclaim our original birthright to reach our full potential.

I'd like to pose this question to you: Would you rather adhere to fears and limitations or respond to the deep, burning desire within you to take up space and actualize your dreams? The reality is that burning desire won't go away. In fact, it'll get louder and peskier the more you try to stifle it. Is there a risk in living out loud? Yes. But if you remain a shell of who you are, how can you open yourself up to the people, places, and opportunities that are waiting for the best version of you? I'm not going to pretend that showing up as your full, authentic self in this world is completely safe at this moment in time. But simply seeing yourself fully as a Black woman is a revolutionary act that builds your confidence and sense of self. You can begin working through your fears of success by taking note of your own behaviors. Ask yourself these questions:

- When I'm scrolling on social media, do I find myself being quick to judge someone sharing a hard-earned accomplishment? Am I critical if I often see them post good news, even if they are transparent about the ups and downs along the way? Why is that? Keep in mind that no one owes the public access to their difficult times in order to be deemed worthy of success.

- Am I projecting my own limiting beliefs on someone else, which is ultimately hurting me? Remember: the critical eye with which you view others is the same one that you use on yourself. If you can stop judging others harshly and resist the urge to critique or "knock them down a peg," you will be kinder to yourself as well.

- Imagine how much freer you'll feel if you allow yourself to try something new, grow, and be successful without the fear of *What will other people think? Will they think I'm trying to be better than them?*

- I invite you to explore the following: Whose judgment do you fear if you succeed? Do you think they'll be critical of what you did to get there (e.g., setting more boundaries, having a more demanding schedule, etc.)? How can you begin to allow yourself to savor your success and not shy away from it or sabotage it?

AIM TO BE KIND, NOT NICE

The kind of self-sacrifice required to be nice is killing women, especially Black women. Repressed emotions have been linked to higher rates of autoimmune disorders and undiagnosable mystery symptoms among Black women.[1] So it's important, to say

---

1   Maytal Eyal, "Self-Silencing Is Making Women Sick," *Time*, October 3, 2023, https://time.com/6319549/silencing-women-sick-essay.

the least, for you to release yourself from the shackles of being perceived as "good" in everyone's eyes. I know how deeply we've been conditioned to care more about other people and how our actions might impact them than ourselves. We've been brought up in homes where we saw how girls were treated differently from their brothers, we've attended church and felt uncomfortable in our own skin because our naturally developing bodies were believed to be at fault for the waywardness of men's eyes, and we can't just walk down the street feeling whatever we're feeling without being told to smile. The list goes on and on. We collected evidence early in life that we should be overly concerned with how we are viewed. And these experiences added up over time to create deeply held beliefs that it is our job to ensure everyone feels happy and approves of each decision we make, which is an impossible task, not to mention that our own happiness is sacrificed in the process.

When we come to this realization, we must decide whether we want to continue placating others at the expense of our own dreams and success or make the uncomfortable decision to prioritize our needs and thereby risk being seen as unkind or, even more common, as a b*+@#. Which will you choose?

To be transparent, it has been extremely hard for me at times to make decisions that have made me seem mean or not nice—not just because of the internal work I needed to do to feel okay with how others perceived me, but also because the nature of this work involves giving, serving, and caring for people. This can create an even greater expectation for me to appease and fully give of myself to others. People sometimes associate kindness with weakness, and that assumption has opened me up to various traumatic experiences that one wouldn't think I'd be exposed to since I created this company, but unfortunately, I have been. My words and work have been copied and stolen (with the added blow of having that stolen work recognized by bigger platforms—ouch!), I've experienced gaslighting and manipulation from people I hired, and I've endured much disappointment, betrayal, trauma, and heartache on the road to manifesting my dreams. Genuinely operating from a kind, concerned, caring, and honest—albeit not perfect—place in a society where manipulation, greed, and deceit are normalized as part of "getting ahead" is often seen as weak. I had to learn that the hard way while leading a growing company, and even while writing this book. It took years of learning and getting tired of seeing the same dynamics play out for me to observe the role I played in how I showed up in the world and in this work. My toxic empathy resulted in continuing to employ people well after they had already shown that they couldn't do the job; they took advantage of my understanding nature to come up with explanations that would buy them time. "Being too nice" looked like paying people on my team who were not performing well more than I paid myself because I wanted to be seen as a nice boss who cared for her employees and invested in them. My good intentions ultimately resulted in work not getting accomplished, which was a disservice to both me and the company. I later would realize this is a common occurrence that many female founders have had to overcome while running their businesses.

My desire to be caring and compassionate, to the extent that it overrode my ability to see situations both within and outside our company for what they were, was hard to unlearn. So, take it from me: there will be decisions that you'll need to make on the journey toward accomplishing your dreams that the world would love to make you as a Black woman feel bad about. Releasing unhealthy relationships will be a normal part of your growth and journey—it doesn't have to mean anything other than that the relationship is no longer a good fit for this chapter in your life. Being able to advocate for yourself as you evolve is a normal part of living a thriving life. You don't have the same desires and needs today as you did ten years ago. And though the perception of Black women being overly accommodating is the norm, I am here to remind you that it is imperative that you enforce your boundaries, prioritize your needs, and aim to be kind, not nice.

I would distinguish between being kind versus nice by their underlying intentions. Kindness involves empathy and considering others outside of yourself without abandoning your own needs. Niceness is largely influenced by how other people view our actions, which often requires toxic empathy and an extreme lack of boundaries. You cannot live a life you truly enjoy if others' opinions of you are always at the forefront of your mind.

You will disappoint other people on your life journey. There will be people who will project all of "their stuff" onto you and will not like you, no matter how good and kind you are to them. To this, I say accept this reality. Others may think you're mean simply because you advocate for yourself and make choices that are fair based on facts rather than toxic empathy. That's okay. Your strong sense of self and your trusted community will be your guiding light as you center how you feel about yourself

rather than the muck of others' ill-informed opinions and judgments. You will need to rely on your inner compass, your sense
of self-worth, and people who truly know and support you as you
navigate this path. We've seen how Black women's self-advocacy
is often weaponized against them. Black women are viewed negatively when we stand up for ourselves. We are trained to be silent
when someone afflicts us. Instead of recognizing the wrong done
against us, society would have us censor ourselves to be cordial
and "nice." And I would be remiss if I didn't point out that many
are using this phenomenon to their advantage by keeping us Black
women small. But in order for us to take up more space and give
ourselves the opportunity to finally thrive, we have to take the
risk of not being liked.

SMALL, EVERYDAY JOYS AND FREEDOMS

Living your best life isn't just about reaching some lofty goal.
Your best life begins when you decide to make the most of the
very moment you find yourself in right now. This is the magic of
a life well lived. It's a life that doesn't require the perfect conditions for you to find enjoyment and peace, a life in which you can
find a certain level of contentment in the middle of the process.
When you live life this way, you can make room for more of the
blessings you've been praying and sowing for.

So how do you cultivate the kind of life where you can enjoy
the small, everyday moments? Start by engaging your senses and
becoming more present in your day-to-day activities. Driving to
work? Remove the monotony from the task by taking notice of

what you see along the route. *Oh look—the trees are turning colors! The sky has a purple hue to it this morning. It smells like it's about to rain!* This may seem inconsequential, but you're actually training your brain to be more in the present moment rather than letting life pass you by. Make space for mindfulness while you eat. Decide not to use your phone during your lunch break so you can truly focus on the flavors that land on your tongue and how having a good meal and a full belly make you feel. *Safe and comforted? Grateful?* Now that you've savored that feeling of being safe, comforted, and taken care of, how can you translate that feeling to other areas of your life? You'll have a clearer sense of how to create more of those moments and be better able to recognize when you're in environments, spaces, and places that nurture you rather than drain your energy.

Although our society often equates wellness with a certain lifestyle—and you have every right to cultivate whatever lifestyle you wish, sis—there is power in indulging in simple joys that are already available to us but can easily be taken for granted, like fresh air, a walk in the park, basking in the sunshine, drinking clean water, and taking thirty seconds to pause and check in with your breath and how your body feels. Allowing your body to be present and take up space—rather than always existing in fight-or-flight mode—is true freedom. We deserve to harness and cultivate this freedom for ourselves and in community while we await the opportunity to be fully free out in the world.

OUR CALL TO ACTION

My vision and hope for an ideal world in which Black women aren't dying prematurely ground me in this work. I dream of a society in which we, Black women, are fully seen, heard, and loved—not just by ourselves but by our wider community and the world. I don't want us to be loved simply for the physical features and mannerisms that are captured and celebrated by pop culture but are often disdained in our day-to-day lives; I want us to experience love in our rawest, most unadulterated form.

Once black girls breathing® reaches our goal of impacting one million Black women and girls, my hope is that the progress won't end there. My hope is that this work impacts generations to come—providing us with the tools to experience inner peace and freedom, even if we don't experience full freedom in the outside world in my lifetime. I have done the work I felt called to do and planted seeds that will bear fruit in another space and lifetime.

It's important for each of us as Black women to work with what we have in this very moment. We may not yet have all the tools we need to reach our goals, but we need to ask ourselves this: What internal work will we commit to so that the next generation can take this healing and equality work a step further? Specifically—reader, what will *you* do? We need to start by both acknowledging the lack of freedom we see, feel, and experience in our external realities, while also deciding to cultivate freedom within—as our people have always done. Whether our people were singing songs of unity while picking cotton on the plantation or holding hands in prayer at church, we've always known how to create our own safe spaces amidst suffering.

GO-DEEPER EXERCISE: RELEASING THE NEED TO BE NICE

Take some time to reflect on the following prompts. As you sit with your answers, notice what feelings come up for you and what sensations arise in your body.

- Recall a time when you allowed others' opinions of you to influence what you did in a way that did not prioritize yourself or your needs. How did the situation play out and how did you end up feeling?
- When you think about not being liked, whether by specific individuals or a group, what feelings come up for you? How have you tried to avoid situations in which people might have an unfavorable opinion of you?
- Who will you need to be in order to fulfill your dreams? In what ways will you need to show up in the world? How does that differ from how you show up now?
- Who do you admire for their courage to risk not being liked in order to fulfill their destiny? How can their story encourage you in triggering times?

ENVISIONING EXERCISE

Close your eyes and get settled into a comfortable position. Turn your attention to your natural breathing pattern, noticing and tapping in to your inhales and exhales. Picture yourself in the world accomplishing your dreams while making difficult decisions about who you need to be to make those dreams a reality. Allow your inhales and exhales to deepen as you picture that version of yourself.

What affirmative words would you tell that version of yourself to let her know that she is safe and worthy of making choices that prioritize her own dreams and needs?

What sense of comfort does she need to feel in her body? How can you offer yourself that comfort in your physical body right now? Maybe it's a big hug, or gently rocking your body from left to right as one would comfort a baby. Whatever the motion, give that to yourself.

Think about all the people in your life who know you and your character and will be there to support you in challenging times. Now picture yourself walking through a period when you are not liked for making a decision that was in your best interest. Declare affirmations over that version of yourself. Offer her physical comfort. See her supportive tribe gather around her. Tell your future self that you're so excited about who she will become by being brave enough to risk her likability and invest in her dreams.

Conclusion

UNTIL WE BREATHE TOGETHER AGAIN

YOU MAY HAVE experienced many emotions as you turned the pages of this book and dove into the exercises, and I want to validate all your emotions. Sadness, anger, grief, joy, and hopefully a few chuckles here and there. I want to personally thank you for taking the time to invest in yourself and your healing. For when you heal yourself, you heal and impact those around you. My prayer is that every Black woman who is tired, emotionally drained, hopeless, in despair, or lonely gets to encounter the powerful resources and reflections shared in this book at some point in her life because they are life-changing. My purpose and mission with this work began with me healing myself and daring to experience life in the fullness of all it could be. To show up bold and Black in each room that God afforded me.

I hope, as I've reached heights with this work that I never could have fathomed, that it makes the journey of those who come after me a little less rough. I hope my sacrifices and hard work are not in vain, but that through those learnings, the Black women witnessing my journey and reading these words will gain something useful for their own paths—healing their bodies, combatting chronic stress, and addressing the traumas that have kept us from thriving.

After you've sat with the emotions and insights that have come from this book, go forth, Black girl. Know that you have everything you need housed in your bones to create the life that you desire. Know that the resistance you exhibit in doing something as intuitive yet intentional as taking a deep breath is demonstrating a kind of care and prioritization of self that our ancestors dreamed of. Don't let your work and healing journey stop there. Continue this revolution with us by becoming one of One Million Black Women taking one step further in improving their health, and #takethepledge by visiting our website at blackgirlsbreathing .com, where you can download your free mental health tool kit. As always, you are most welcome to commune with us in deeper healing work and sisterhood by joining our sunday balm® community (visit app.blackgirlsbreathing.com). I love you, sis. Thank you. Thank you. Thank you.

To every Black girl breathing, always remember: this joy we have—the world didn't give it, and the world will never take it away.

ACKNOWLEDGMENTS

God, thank you. Thank you for permitting me the opportunity to share these words with the world. I was always meant to write this book, and in spite of the many challenges along the way, with your help, I channeled the wisdom you afforded me and I made it happen. Thank you for instilling this mission and dream within me, in spite of my initial resistance, and showing me that through you all things are possible. Thank you for replenishing my hope to keep pushing to see it come to pass. Thank you for renewing my strength during the valleys of this journey. And I want to thank myself for being obedient to your call, for "obedience is better than sacrifice" (1 Samuel 15:22).

Mom, thank you for being my biggest cheerleader and best friend. Thank you for the scriptures every morning and for supporting my vision. For allowing me to come over without much advance notice and for always responding with excitement when I call and tell you I'm on my way. Thank you for your sacrifices that have impacted our entire family. For being an example of what it means to honor your bloodline by taking on the role of being a full-time caregiver and for being a Renaissance woman in all that you are and have accomplished. I'm grateful to have witnessed that growing up, and I'm in awe of how you balanced it all.

Dad, thanks for investing in the dance lessons and extracurricular activities over the years. They weren't in vain. Thank you for exposing me to Black excellence and gifting me with your knack for math and science. I'm putting them to good use now.

Grandma Kate, thank you for being brave enough to leave Money, Mississippi, that day. I know I get some of my fighter spirit from you. And thank you for running into James Howell and marrying him. Grandpa (Paw Paw), I wish you were here to see this. I know it'd make you so proud. Thank you for being the first to defend and affirm my boldness and defiance early on. It has shaped who I am today. Thank you for the sacrifices you made that still impact our family. I love you and miss you so much. Spending extensive time with you and Grandma Kate has been such an immense honor.

Grandma and Grandpa Clark, I hope when you look down from Heaven, any sacrifice you made in raising your family feels like it was well worth it. I hope you're proud.

To my brother and sister, Jamison and Lauren: love you both.

Thank you to the rest of my extended family. You make me proud to be a part of your bloodline. To those who now watch us from Heaven: we miss you greatly, and I vow to live each day as the gift it is.

To my dear sistah- and brotha-friends: Thank you for being my chosen family and a safe space for me to land. Special shout-out to those of you who thought the most of me and encouraged me while I had my head down working on this book. You know who you are!

To all the Black women who've ever supported me along my journey, listened to my words, written me, and encouraged me to keep going: You're the reason why I continue to do what I do. I'm honored to serve you with this work. To one million and beyond!

Joanna Ng, thank you for further editing my words to perfection.

Thank you to my body for carrying me through. We've been through so much during the creation of this book. Thank you for showing me that you're stronger than I ever realized. Thank you for helping me to create the boundaries needed to keep showing up in the world.

And to my younger self—see? It all worked out, and is working out, for your good. To my future self: I hope you're worrying a lot less and enjoying the fruits of my current labor.

And in the vein of "writing the vision and making it plain," to my future husband and children: I hope I make you proud.

INDEX

Index

ABOUT THE AUTHOR

Jasmine Marie is a speaker, breathwork practitioner, and the CEO and founder of black girls breathing.® She is driven by a commitment to improve health outcomes for underserved communities and Black women specifically. Her innovative vision and execution to provide accessible wellness and somatic health tools to heal trauma and decrease chronic stress have impacted tens of thousands of Black women to date, with a mission to impact over one million with her work. She has made history introducing this work to new platforms and audiences. Further demonstrating her breadth of expertise and experience, she has shared her professional wisdom to a range of demographics—from a juvenile detention center to Ivy League colleges and Fortune 100 companies. She has been featured on *Good Morning America*, and in premier publications including *O, the Oprah Magazine*, *Vogue*, *Forbes*, *Harper's Bazaar*, *Marie Claire*, *Essence*, *Nylon*, *Black Enterprise*, and the *Wall Street Journal*, among others. Marie is a graduate of the NYU Stern School of Business and is a serial entrepreneur with a corporate professional background in global brand management. She is a proud Atlanta native.

To further connect with her and learn more about her work, visit thejasminemarie.com and blackgirlsbreathing.com.